Gary Pickler

ENERGY TOOLS
By Gary Pickler

Lulu

2022

ENERGY TOOLS.

Disclaimer. This book is not intended as medical advice. Its intent is solely informational and educational. Please, consult a health professional if you have questions about your health. The author and publisher are not liable for any damages or negative consequences from any treatment, action, application, or preparation, to any person reading or following the information in this book.

First edition	: Oct 14, 2022
Editing, page design, proofreading	: Bruno Curfs
	Gary Pickler
Cover design	: Gary Pickler
	Bruno Curfs
	killercovers.com
Author and publisher, through Lulu	: Gary Pickler

Table of Contents

Dedication

This book is dedicated to Fredric Schiffer M.D. and his brilliant, ingenious, and revolutionary science of Dual-Brain Psychology, which he clearly explains in his book "Of Two Minds". Schiffer conclusively proves that the two hemispheres of our brain are really two separate personalities that absolutely must learn to work together as a team if any happiness or success in life is to be attained! (In Energy Tool #31, I will explain more.) Only by reading this incredible book five times, and working with its cutting-edge ideas and methods extensively, was I able to write and finish my book. This is because one hemispheric personality of mine extremely wanted to write this book, but the other hemispheric personality utterly did not!

Please think about the profound significance of this. How can one of your two hemispheric personalities attain any of its life goals, if the other hemispheric personality is continually sabotaging these goals with its own opposite agenda? Incidentally, this is not the Freudian Ego and Id scenario exactly, because Dr. Schiffer clearly shows that both hemispheric personalities are operating consciously (but alternately) in us. It is also not the "inner child" scenario, because the more "childish" hemispheric personality is actively making very consequential life decisions for us, half the time!

If Dr. Schiffer's Dual Brain Psychology is recognized and embraced enough to replace (or at least supplement) the 100-years old antiquated Freudian and Jungian psychologies, this could unify into compatibility the two hemispheric personalities of great numbers of people on our planet, which could very healthily change the destiny of the human race. Be sure to read his book, and successfully apply it in your own life!

Dr. Schiffer invented another very useful tool, called "Schiffer goggles" (available to purchase on the internet). These amazing goggles, when put on, enable you to experience the significant differences (in emotions and attitudes) of your two hemispheric personalities, which then motivates you to begin undertaking a process of communicating and "talking things out" more, between these two completely-different-and-opposite hemispheric personalities. Consider investigating all this further. You'll be very glad that you did!

Introduction

No Stone Has Been Left Unturned Here!

I've done my best to approach the issue of giving you more energy, from *every conceivable angle*! The most nutritious, energy-producing foods, superfoods, energizing vitamins, energizing minerals, energizing herbs, energizing mushrooms, and energizing probiotics are explained in depth. Energizing Chinese Medicine tools, American Indian tools, shamanic tools, massage tools, reflexology tools, aerobics tools, power-dance tools, yoga tools, and energy-giving breathing tools are disclosed. Energy tools involving lymph, sweating, naps, meditation, and aromatherapy are revealed.

Unusual energizing "apparatus-contraption-device" tools like the Back-Roller-Massager and Theracane (to give you "back heaven"), mini-rebounder, power rocking chair, and enema hose, are divulged.

Energizing crystals, water therapy, sunlight power, chi-energy, reversed moonlight power, and color therapy tools are uncovered and unmasked.

Energizing psychological and inspiring methods, never seen before, are included here. Clearly shown here are energy tools that explain what to avoid that decreases your energy!

And lastly, there are energy tools, brought to light, that will utterly blow your mind, besides recharging your body, with enormous revitalizing re-energization!

All-in-all, there are 101 totally different energy tools here, all explained fully in detail. After familiarizing yourself with them all, take your pick! Choose one (or more) of the 101 methods that really seems to fit you and your unique style of energizing yourself. Then, do these energy tools. And, finally be a lot more full of energy, to start living the happy, successful, cured-from-fatigue life that you've always wanted, deep down in your soul!

Why I Wrote This Book For You And Others

I feel enormous compassion for all those struggling with exhaustion and fatigue. It's because of these deep feelings that I want so much to help. So I'm very motivated to make a difference, however much I can, with this book of Energy Tools.

Over many decades I've known several dozen people who miraculously overcame their fatigue to generate a lot more energy. When I questioned them as to *how*, they all freely confided their techniques to me. In this way, I gradually collected several dozen Energy Tools over time. Eventually, I knew it was finally time to write this book.

I sincerely hope this book makes a difference to you and others in the world. May it greatly help all those needing energy-increasing tools. This book is dedicated to all people in the world who would appreciate having more energy in their daily life.

From the bottom of my heart, I offer this book to you, to nurture and empower you to have more energy. May it greatly help you to energetically heal and change your life, so that you'll be happier and more successful.

Even if only *one* person in the world uses this book to more effectively increase their energy, it will be a success.

God Bless!
Gary Pickler
Energy Tool Healer

Energy Tools #1 - #101

The Energy Tools are alphabetically ordered, and also numbered.

Energy Tool

#1. Acupressure Points Of Power

There is an acupressure point, called the "three more miles"-point, that gives you a *burst of energy*, when pressed! It has its name because in ancient China, it enabled an exhausted person to walk three more miles!

This energy-producing point is located just below both knobs of the knee (the higher big knob, and the lower smaller knob), on the *outside* of your shin bone. In other words, your knee has two knobs in front. There's the relatively big "upper knob", i.e., the knee disc (*patella*). About 3 inches below this, there is a smaller "lower knob", i.e., the top of the shin bone (*tibia*). Press about 1 inch below the "lower knob", and 1 inch to the *outside* of the shin bone (the bone that runs down from this "lower knob" to your ankle).

Obviously, press this point under both the right and left knee. Press this point as hard as you can (without hurting yourself too much). As you press in with your fingers, circle your fingers around a little, as you press in. You'll find this gives you a burst of energy!

Also, the military recommends another point to press, that gives you a burst of energy. This "hand point" is at the very bottom of the "V" between your thumb and index finger. In fact, this point is about two inches below where the skin ends. Press very, very hard on this point, pinching from both sides of your hand, on this hand point, to make it work! When I've tried this and pressed extremely hard, it has worked and given me an energy burst! Press this "V"-point on both right and left hands.

Try combining the knee points and hand points, along with pressing a *third* energy point hard, just under the middle of the nose (on your extreme upper lip). This should give you a big triple burst of energy when needed!

Energy Tool

#2. Aerobic Shape

Several friends of mine, who used to have trouble with low energy, told me that once they got in aerobic shape, they "waved their fatigue goodbye". This is because energy is very connected with our endocrine system and bodily organs. Just look at children and all the other mammals. Notice how energetic they are and how their energy is very connected to the movements and activities of their body, as they rapidly and actively move about!

But you *must* exercise aerobically with an activity that you *really like*! This is ultra-important! Otherwise, the odds are that you *just won't stick with it*. Why should you, if a type of activity bores you, or you just *don't like it*?

Compile a list of 100 different ways to exercise, using the internet. You'll be *amazed* at how many ways there are to get in aerobic shape! Then, put a (1), (2), and (3) by your top three choices. These (1), (2), and (3) should be the ways that are the *most fun* for you! So, these activities will then be what works for you!

Of course, if it turns out that *none* of these 100 ways of exercising appeal to you, then joining a gym may be necessary. Then, when you arrive at the gym and see everyone else exercising, you'll be motivated by simple "crowd psychology" to join in!

Anyway, give "aerobic shape exercising" a chance, to energize yourself and greatly reduce any fatigue!

Energy Tool

#3. Air Filter In Home

- If you live in a polluted area where the air is bad, your energy can be improved by filtering out the 450 or so environmental toxins present in bad air. You'll be surprised how much better and more energetic you'll feel, with *better air* to breathe!

- Get on the internet and research how you can greatly improve the quality of air in your home, car, and possibly even workplace.

- Since high-quality oxygen (without environmental toxins) is greatly needed to fire-up all your cellular reactions (that produce your energy), you can see the ultra-importance here, of quality air.

- Start making quality air your top priority!

Energy Tool

#4. Alcohol – Minimize Or Stop It

Everyone already knows that too much alcohol is bad for one's health. Yet, it's so hard to stop or even cut down. Well, I've written another book, available from Lulu.com, entitled *Stop Alcohol Fast – 55 Methods That Actually Work* by Gary Pickler.

This book really does the job and will definitely stop or cut down your alcohol. Buy it, if you want results!

Energy Tool

#5. Ally/Sub-Self Method

No matter how much our society gives us the idea that we are "one", instead, really we are "many". That is, every one of us has many different parts that can be called "sub-selves", "sub-personalities", "characters", "archetypes" (in Jungian psychology), or "allies" (in the Carlos Castanada series of "Don Juan" books).

Start off by making a list of all your different parts. You probably have a worker, a player, a social communicator/social actor part, a bossy part, a romantic part, a loyal friend part, an internalized father/mother part (Freud's "Superego"), and a depressed, angry, fearful, upset child part (Freud's "Id"). Also, Jung's archetypes of "Shadow", "Trickster", and "Hero/Warrior/Savior" are probably in the mix, too. Is there also a lazy part, or a goof-off part, along with a comedian? Already that's 14 if you have them all. Do you see what I mean, how ultra-complex we all are?

Now, examine all your sub-selves and find perhaps the three strongest, who really want to help you to become more energized. Perhaps they would be three of these four: the *Superego*, the *Hero/Warrior/Savior*, the *bossy* part, or the *Worker*.

So now, when you've chosen your strongest sub-selves, all with strong willpower to help you to become more energized, draw all their faces! Using colored pencils or even crayons, use your intuition to draw their faces, either on white card stock, or on 8-1/2 × 11 printer paper.

If you're new to this "intuitive drawing" or "drawing from your subconscious", take your time. But, try to intuitively "channel" three or four drawings. Take three or four days, or even a week, if you need to.

These three or four drawings of your strongest sub-selves are now your allies! And, by talking to, and calling on these allies to help you, they'll often respond to help you increase your energy.

Call on the *strength* of these allies as you look at their faces that you've drawn. Ask, beseech, or even *command* them to help you! Perhaps say, "All right, already, all you guys! You're the toughest dudes I've got in this psyche of mine! Well, let's stop this darn fatigue problem! Enough, already! Let's have some *power* to *totally knock off* this low-energy *bullshit* that's wrecking our life! Come on! Let's do it, you guys! I know you have the *power* to make it happen, so let's go! Yeah! Let's do it! Start energizing me! Now!!!

Obviously, everyone will have their own style of talking to their strongest allies. So, do all this in *your own way*! Perhaps, also, these allies can increase your energy by getting into *their* favorite activity instead.

Energy Tool

#6. Aromatherapies That Energize Will Power

I've found that these three aromatherapies: 1.) pine, 2.) basil, and 3.) patchouli, give me energy and willpower to propel me into action, to *get the job done*! These three aromatherapies call up reserves of energy to "make things happen"! (You can experiment with other aromatherapies, too, to see which ones energize you the most.)

Bach flower remedies or other flower essences might do the energizing job for you here too. Anyway, try pine, basil, and patchouli, and see if they energetically work for you too!

Energy Tool

#7. Art Project Initiate

We all know how much energy kids have when they're running around and playing creative games. Very natural moving, singing, dancing, and creativity occur spontaneously when we're in this more child-like state. Right? In fact, art and music projects tend to put us in these more energetic child-like states, when we've creatively engaged. Haven't you noticed?

One of the reasons for this is that our "inner child" can get really *bored* from a "grown-up life" of work and chore-doing. This boredom can lead to depression, from the sheer lack of fun. Eventually, our "inner child" even starts to "hibernate" inside us, and energy levels can plummet!

The creative fun of art and music breaks this "depressed-hybernation" cycle, to re-awaken our inner, magical child, once again! A great energizing occurs when suddenly, our inner child can come out and play again! So, energize yourself by treating yourself to plenty of art, music, and fun, whenever you feel you really need it. Fill yourself with energy through the exciting, fun creativity of your inner child, on a regular basis!

Energy Tool

#8. B-Vitamin Energy

Taking a daily B-vitamin really helps to give your body more energy. But because all the B-vitamins work together as a "team", all eleven B-vitamins are necessary.

Vitamins B1 (thiamin), B2 (riboflavin), B3 (niacin or niacinamide as a better form), choline (formerly B4), B5 (pantothenic acid), B6 (pyridoxine, pyridoxal, or pyridoxamine), B7 (biotin), B8 (inositol), B9 (folic acid), B10 (PABA or para-amino-benzoic acid), and B12 (cobalamins, such as cyanocobalamin) are *all* necessary to be present in the vitamin B complex.

If even *one* (of these eleven B vitamins) is missing, then find another brand of vitamin B complex, with all these eleven B-vitamins in it. This is very, very important! If you neglect this, and if even *one* B-vitamin is missing, then you'll gradually become deficient in the missing B-vitamin, and the whole remedy will be wrecked. Deficiency in the missing B-vitamin usually causes a type of "unexplained fatigue", I've found from experience.

Also, the vitamin B3 in the B complex capsule needs to be vitamin B3 in the form of niacinamide and not niacin. This is because vitamin B3 as niacin causes an itchy, red, unpleasant flush in the face and all over the body. To prevent this extreme flushing irritation, vitamin B3 as niacinamide (and not niacin) should be taken.

A good brand of multiple B vitamins, for a very reasonable price, is Solaray B-Complex 50, in a 50 capsule bottle. It can be ordered at

- http://www.solaray.com/

or by phoning 1 (800) 683-9640.

Solaray B-complex 50 is highly recommended, since it has all the above requirements and is inexpensive!

Often people are deficient in one or more of these B-vitamins, without even knowing it.

Anyway, you should feel the extra energy in your body, once you start taking (daily) a capsule of these ultra-important B-vitamins!

Energy Tool

#9. Back Roller Massager (Or Theracane)

(Gives you "Back Heaven".)

There is a very effective way to massage your back by yourself, with the following tool! I invented it, and it's called (by me) either a *Back Roller Massager*, or a *BlissR*. This is how you (fairly easily) make it:

(1) Buy a wood rod (called a "dowell") at the hardware store or Home Depot, etc., of 5/8 inch diameter. Usually these dowells are about 3 or 4 feet long.

(2) Saw off a 15-inch length of this dowell, to use in making this tool. File smooth the ends of your 15-inch wood rod. Then, mark (with a pen) a circle around the exact middle of your 15-inch rod. Obviously, this circle will be 7 1/2 inches in, from each end of the rod.

(3) Buy 2 "Pinky Balls" on the internet (do a search for "Pinky Balls"). Or you could possibly use heavy-duty tennis balls, perhaps bought at Walmart, but they won't be as pleasurable as Pinky Balls. The diameter of the Pinky Balls should be about 2 1/4 inches (they're approximately the same size as tennis balls).

(4) Get ready to drill a 5/8 inch diameter hole halfway through a spot you mark on a Pinky Ball. First, mark the spot with a pen. Then, using a measuring tape (or a ruler that you precisely roll around the ball's curvature) find the exact point on the ball that is exactly 180 degrees opposite the first spot. This is the hardest part, in measuring very, very carefully to find this "opposite point". If the second point (to be drilled) is not precisely located, then the ball will "wobble" too much on the rod, when used later. The best method here is to start by marking the spot where the first hole is to be drilled. Then, measuring around the ball (both horizontally and vertically) accurately locate the point on the ball exactly 180 degrees opposite the first spot. Next, drill a 5/8 inch diameter hole only halfway through the Pinky Ball, from the first spot. Then, drill another 5/8 inch hole through the second point. Halfway through the ball, your drill should enter the "void" caused by the first drilling (which was only halfway through), and then you've gotten the needed hole, completely through the ball.

(5) Drill a 5/8 inch hole through the second Pinky Ball, in exactly the same way as with the first Pinky Ball.

(6) Once the (exactly opposite) holes are drilled, insert the 15-inch

rod through both balls. The balls should end up about 1 1/2 inches away from the center circle that you marked on the rod in step (2). Thus, the 2 Pinky Balls are positioned on the rod 3 inches apart, in the best location. They'll be massaging your back, on either side of your spine.

(7) So now, place the Back Roller Massager between your back and a wall (or your front door, or the side of a stable bookcase). Carefully lean back against the 2 balls of the Back Roller Massager (while standing), with the 2 balls on either side of your spine. Bend your knees more, then less, etc., to result in the moving of your back up and down against the wall, while your back pleasurably presses into the 2 balls. Doesn't this make your back feel really good? You'll probably need to practice a bit to get the hang of this! You'll also need to keep re-positioning the Back Roller Massager, with your hands, by reaching around behind you.

(8) Later on, try adding little screws (or screwed-on pieces of wood) to either side of the 2 balls. This will help keep the 2 balls in place; it stops them from shifting around so much when in use and occasionally needing adjustment.

(9) Still later on, you can try adding 2 looped slim ropes to either side of the balls. These ropes loop around the outer edges of the rod, and go (from behind you) to drape over your shoulders, then come down to where your hands can grab them. Your hands can then pull on these ropes, to adjust the position of the 2 balls, up and down on your back, to either side of your spine.

(10) Practice with this tool until you get quite skillful with it, then regularly massage your back daily to achieve "back heaven". Yes! Your back will feel absolutely incredible from this daily "back bliss". Also, your energy will then noticeably increase, when you've facilitated a very healthy back and spine!

Theracane "Nirvana"

There is another incredible back-massaging tool on the internet called a theracane. It's shaped like a sickle, and curves around to pleasurably massage your back, as you hold it.

I bought one on Amazon.com for $29 (free shipping). It's amazing, and also gives enormous "back heaven". (Don't be tempted by any inferior "cheap imitations", but get the genuine theracane, here, to unerringly get your daily "back bliss".)

Energy Tool

#10. Bad-Back Exercises

There are nine simple exercises that stretch and move your back in unique ways, so that your back feels superb! Any pain in your back will stop or be reduced. Your posture will spontaneously improve, your breathing will naturally deepen, and you'll resultantly have more energy!

Directions on doing the nine simple bad-back exercises (that should only take 5 minutes total, once you learn them):

1. Do the "twist" (Rock & Roll 1960s Dance). Stand, and gently swing your arms and shoulders to the right, as simultaneously you swing your hips to the left (opposite direction). Then "reverse-swing" this, and gently swing your arms and shoulders to the left, as simultaneously you swing your hips to the right (opposite direction). Keep doing this "twisting" motion, several times. It really stretches your back!

2. Still standing, move your belly button point in a circle (about one foot in diameter), parallel to the floor. In other words, swing your mid-section and belly button around in a circle, first clockwise for perhaps 4 times, then counterclockwise 4 times.

3. Still standing, face a bare wall (or closed door). Now, move your belly button in a one-foot diameter circle that's parallel to the wall. To do this, you'll need to rise up on your toes to make the high curve of the circle, then bend your knees a little, to make the lower curve of the circle. Do clockwise 4 times, then counterclockwise 4 times.

4. Still standing, move your belly button in a one-foot circle in the last of 3 dimensions! This circle will be parallel to the walls on either side of you. To make it, you'll need to move your body forward, then rise-on-your-toes upward and back, then move back behind you, then (bending your knees) go low and back to where you started. Do 4 times in this forward direction, then 4 times in the reverse direction of all this.

And now, for 5, 6, 7, and 8, you'll need to kneel (on padding?) on the floor, then lean forward to place your hands on the floor, about shoulder-width apart. This is the position in which people used to do "knee push-ups" (push-ups done on your knees, instead of on your toes). But we won't be doing any push-ups, here, in this position.

5. In this "knee push-up" position, and by using your back muscles as much as possible (instead of your arms) move your upper body forward, then your upper body down low, then

draw your upper body back (still down low), then move your upper body back up again, returning to the start. In other words, you're sort of making a circular movement of your upper body: forward, down, down and back, up, return to start. Do this 4 times. Then do the exact reverse of this 4 times (using the same circular motion, but in reverse).

6. In the "knee push-up" position, "look at your heels". First, swing your head and upper body out to the right, so that you can look at your right heel. Do 4 times (back and forth) to the right. Then, do 4 times (back and forth) to the left, looking at the left heel.

7. Putting all your lower body's weight on your left knee, put your right knee up against your chest. Then, go ahead and stretch your right leg back straight, behind you. Then do the left leg similarly. In alternating with the legs, do each leg 4 times.

8. "Point to the ceiling" with your right hand, then your left hand, alternately. To do this, you'll have to twist your upper body up to right, then up to left. Do 4 times, right and left. Go, with your hands, up as high as you can, knowing that you'll improve on this, with practice.

9. Lie on your back, with your legs pointing straight up. Slowly move your legs about 12 inches forward, then back, several times. Feel the slight stretching in your lower back.

Okay, that's it! Your back is much more stretched, and you should feel more energized now!

Energy Tool

#11. Biorhythms

When I experimented with biorhythms, I calculated (for the month) my intellectual high, low, and critical days; my emotional high, low, and critical days; and my physical high, low, and critical days. It seemed to work. I could actually feel the energies that the biorhythm book said I should feel, on those days! (But possibly not everyone will be able to "tune in", and feel the reality of all this, too.)

At any rate, by knowing in advance how you'll feel mentally, physically, and emotionally on future days (your "internal weather", so to speak) this foreknowledge can be put to good use in managing your energy! You can schedule future work and projects based on future energy predictions. (Or avoid scheduling them, if a future day happens to be a "downer".)

You'll need to experiment with all this, obviously. Buy a biorhythms book on the internet, and begin to find out whether your future days approximately occur as predicted. If it (sort of) works, and you're a boss, try it also on the workers under you, to facilitate their best performance, too.

So, check out biorhythms, if you desire the power-knowledge of future energizations that it can provide for you!

Note. If you fail to explore biorhythms, but your rivals do instead, then you could greatly be taken advantage of in the future, when your rivals schedule confrontations on your "baddest" day! (For example, a "triple low" day, when you're mentally, emotionally, and physically lowest, all at the same time!)

P.S. A shortcut, for experimentation, here, is to find out the day of the week that you were born. Well, whatever that day is, you will repeatedly have (for life) either an emotionally critical day, or an emotionally low day, or an emotionally high day, on that very day. For example, if you were born on a Friday, then every Friday (for life!) will be emotionally "challenging". So, the experimental shortcut, here, is to find out the day of the week that you were born on, and with reflective open-mindedness, see if that particular day of the week has always been a bit "emotionally challenging". Has it been? Well, if it has been, then this must mean that biorhythms definitely work, for you, and it will become very energetically powerful for you to explore and use biorhythms in the future, before your opponents, rivals, and even enemies begin using it—disastrously—against you!

Energy Tool

#12. Book Of Internal Exercises

Stephen T. Chang wrote a book in 1978 entitled "The Book of Internal Exercises". Based on powerful energizing techniques from 6,000-years-old Chinese medicine, the dozens of exercises in this book will energize you beyond your wildest dreams!

All that's needed (to abundantly energize your entire body, through doing many of the exercises in this book) is the self-discipline to do, daily, a hand-picked selection of the energizing exercises!

It really works. Try it!

P.S. Brushing your hands along the 14 energy meridians (guiding yourself by acupuncture point charts from the internet) works very well, too. Also, getting a practitioner's acupressure massage or shiatsu massage energizes you quite a bit. This can motivate you to learn these two types of massage yourself, to then do regularly on yourself!

P.P.S. Mantak Chia wrote many books full of very energizing exercises (from Chinese medicine). I strongly recommend Mantak Chia's "Chi Self-Massage" and "Taoist Ways to Transform Stress Into Vitality".

Energy Tool

#13. Brain Gym Exercises

Brain Gym consists in making dozens of hand and bodily movements that result in both of your brain hemispheres becoming more active and working together. This results in several very good consequences, including being more energized and happy!

There are many books on the internet that fully instruct you in Brain Gym and its many techniques. One book is "Brain Gym and Me", by Paul Dennison, which I've read.

It's highly recommended that you experiment with Brain Gym techniques. This just may result in a very potent form of extreme energization for you, and your two brain hemispheres!

Energy Tool

#14. Brain Relax

The goal of this technique (or process) is to relax, soothe, and bring more peace and calm to a stressed-out, wound-up, rat-race-running brain and ego trying (almost desperately) to survive and thrive, in our "asphalt jungle" American Society (which so often is "dog-eat-dog and rat-eat-rat").

Here's how it works:

- Lie down comfortably on a bed or couch. You may need to wear earplugs or noise-reducing headphones (or both) to block out any bothersome noise that could interfere with your "going deep within" yourself, here.

- Now, systematically relax every part of your body. Focus on relaxing your feet, then legs, then lower body, then upper body, then hands and arms, then neck, then head, then face (including your jaw, mouth, and eyes). You can do this body-relaxing process in any order that you want. To help with this, you can tape record the 172 "relax-relax-relax" words from my book "Stop Smoking Fast", p. 46, or from my book "Stop Alcohol Fast", p. 12, then play this tape recording back to yourself.

- Once your body is extremely relaxed, move your attention to the center of your brain! Get in touch with the "raw" ego-brain energy there, as you compassionately observe it, without judgement. Many people experiencing this center-of-the-brain, "raw" ego energy are (at first) shocked at how intense it is! When I first tried this, it felt like a desperate and cornered rat, or a lizard, or a small animal, caught by a human's hand, struggling frantically to escape and not be killed. I got in touch that our ego is extremely pressured to satisfy all our body's instincts, and also all our society's expectations, almost all the time. How utterly, incredibly stressful this is! We have to earn money, do our chores, take care of our health and body, manage our possessions, deal with the idiosyncrasies of family members and friends (and even strangers), entertain ourselves and others, use fairly good social skills, obey a multitude of customs and laws, engage in spiritual practices (perhaps), release pent-up negativity, have time for art or music, deal with bad luck and accidents, and even try for some recognition or fame (perhaps). What an incredibly tough "juggling act", required of our brain and ego, for living a "full" life! No wonder we're so stressed out (and sometimes even close to a nervous breakdown) from all this!

- Well, when we totally relax our body, then move our compassionate, non-judging, observing attention to the center of our brain, we often experience something like a "hurricane" or "cyclone", there. It can be very shockingly intense, at first. But, try to keep your observing attention there, as you somehow attempt (with some kind of meditative, or "psychic", or focusing, or self-loving, or "letting go", or praying, or "grace-of-God" ability you develop) to soothe or calm it down, bringing more peace to it, little by little. Calm, relaxed, deeper breathing helps. Just totally relax your lungs and breathing (without any effort to breathe in this way), but just by totally relaxing your lungs, to let them breathe naturally, in this extremely relaxed way. You'll find that any peace, calm, and soothingness that you can bring to this "cauldron of ego stress", at the center of your brain, will result in feeling much better. You'll be more calmly energized, after you're done, and ready to come out of this relaxed state to resume your normal life again. Try it! (Being in water, a bathtub, a river, a lake, or the ocean helps a lot when doing this stress-releasing process.)

Energy Tool

#15. Canine Yoga

Dogs do about a dozen things that maintain their energy and psychological health. We can learn from them, and even imitate some of their healthy habits! If this seems a little weird, remember that many T'ai Chi Ch'uan movements originated from the ancient Chinese masters' observations of various animal movements.

Imitating the spontaneous and "wild" behaviors of dogs (all of which affect them physically and emotionally) can be a catalyst that helps us be more "wild" and thus access more energy from our subconscious "id" part. So, experimentally try some of these dog behaviors, and experience an increase in energy from them!

1. Shaking. When dogs feel any weird or upsetting emotions from the environment, they shake (as if they've just come out of the water). Try this! Whenever you're feeling shocked, angry, anxious, etc., try "shaking it off, like a dog". It just might work, and you'll feel better. (If at work, you obviously might need to go do it in a restroom stall, or somewhere else that's private, like your car.)

2. Back Twisting. You may have seen a dog on its back, on the grass, twisting ecstatically back and forth, with extreme enjoyment. Try this (gently, at first) on your bed, or on a pillow on your rug. It makes your back feel "super", once you've practiced it and got the hang of it.

3. Doggie Stretching. You've probably seen a standing dog stretch its front paws out quite a bit, and move its rear end back, as its stomach falls down near the floor, and its head points up a little. The dog looks like it's really enjoying this type of stretch. Try it (gently and carefully, at first)! Obviously, you'll need to get down on a rug, on your hands and knees, to do this one. You won't be sorry!

4. Panting. Try panting like a dog, with your tongue slightly out, and rapidly breathing in and out. Only 10 seconds of this gives you an energizing oxygen rush! And, perhaps it might cool you down, too, either physically or emotionally, or both!

5. Ear petting. Dogs love it when you pet their ears, and pet and rub around their ears. Try it on yourself, to uplevel your mood and feel loved. Really fondle, stroke, and gently play with your ears. Don't forget to gently rub up and down to either side of your ears. It really works, to make you feel better!

6. Howling. Dogs (and coyotes and wolves too) howl out their grief, really effectively! Try this by putting your head and body

completely under the bed covers (so your neighbors won't hear). It really effectively "dispels the blues". Especially after your job, this works well to totally release the day's stresses and unwind, to prepare yourself for some evening fun! Possibly this howling could be done in a shower stall too, as the roaring of full-blast water masks the howling sound.

7. Running side-to-side. Ever notice how a dog (barking at you from behind a fence) will (rapidly and intensely) run from side to side, first to the left, and then to the right, etc.? Try this intense side-to-side running as you look straight ahead, at your (written down) goal. You'll find that it builds up a great emotional eagerness to do this very goal, that you're looking at and focusing upon! From now on, make use of this emotion of "great eagerness", whenever you need it to accomplish any particularly recalcitrant goal of yours. (And, if no one is around watching, you can even add in the ferocious barking, and intense desire to "sink your teeth" into the goal!)

8. Doggy Play. Have you ever seen 2 dogs running around on the grass and (playfully) "nipping" at each other, having great fun? Well, 2 kids (with boffers) or even 2 playful adults (with boffers) can have fun like this, too! (Boffing instead of nipping.)

9. Run around the periphery (of your property, house, work place, or even car). Try doing this "doggie run around the periphery" to get your blood pumping more, and see how much more energized it can make you feel!

10. Biting. Try aggressively biting into pizza, burritos, hamburgers, fries, chips, pasta, gum, fruit, licorice, etc. It very therapeutically releases pent-up jaw tension, plus any "jungle emotions" you're harboring deep within! Wolf it down!

11. Circling around once, twice, or three times before lying down. Many of us have observed this absurd doggie movement that a dog often makes before lying down. Well, if you're willing to experimentally try it yourself before sitting (or lying) down, you just might find that it "mellows you out", or allows you to "let go", as a result of this "circling" type of movement. Try it, see how it alters how you feel, and adopt it, if it works for you. (Be careful of getting overly dizzy and falling down after two or three, or more circles. Perhaps start with just one circle, to safely begin with.)

12. Doggy tug-of-war (as 2 dogs will do, with a toy or bone, etc.). When you and your friend (or relationship partner) are at odds, try a tug-of-war with a rope, kneeling on your living room rug, or standing outside in your yard (or a park). It may need to be "handicapped" to where the woman can use both hands, but

the man can only use one hand (or: 2 women pulling against 1 man). It's excellent for releasing physical aggression, so that the talking-it-out phase, afterward, will be a lot more "civilized". (Also good for 2 kids with "sibling rivalry".)

13. Barking, snarling, and growling. Two people at odds can effectively release aggression by positioning themselves on either side of a fence (like 2 dogs), and loudly barking, snarling, and growling at each other. Let yourself go, and do it to the max! Then, it will be much easier to talk things out later, afterward. (This is also a possible antidote for "nagging" by one partner, since being barked at, snarled at, and growled at is almost funny, and doesn't hurt emotionally like critical, nagging, and cutting words do.)

So, has your "overly civilized" life gone to the dogs? Well, now you know just what to do, Put a bit of healthy, energetic, wildness back into it. Right? Remember: Canine Yoga isn't just for dogs! It just might be something you can really sink your canine teeth into!

Energy Tool

#16. Chi From Hands Into Food

By rubbing your hands together vigorously (for perhaps 10 seconds) you generate "chi", or energy, in your hands! If you then hold the energized chi (in your palms) about 1 inch over any food that you're about to eat, then the palm-chi goes into the food. Shortly afterward, when you chew up and eat this energized food, the energy then goes into your internal organs. Thus, you can energize yourself internally, with this method!

The wise-rascal teacher Gurdjieff expertly used this hand-chi-into-food technique to heal the internal organs of other people, as he energized their insides more, too.

Go slowly with this technique. Energize perhaps only 3 bites of food, at first. Then, gradually increase this process. Your stomach and small intestines aren't used to a lot of energized food, yet. So, expand on this little by little!

Feel the difference, in your stomach, of your hand-energized food going down inside you, to energize your internal organs, more and more. Try it, "vibe it out", and see for yourself its effectiveness!

Energy Tool

#17. Chi From Hands Into Organs

Rub your hands together vigorously (for perhaps 10 seconds) to generate "chi", or energy, in your hands. Then hold the energized chi (in your palms) over any of your organs (or body areas) that you want to be energized!

Holding your chi-energized hands over your navel (belly button) or gut, energizes your intestines and lower body. Or, you can energize your kidneys by reaching your energized hands around behind you. You can energize your liver or gallbladder, or spleen, in the same way. Your energized hands can rub around your chest, in a big circle, to energize your lungs, etc. As you do all this, keep re-energizing your hands periodically, by rubbing them vigorously together (for perhaps 10 seconds) again.

It's not a good idea to hold your energized hands too long, over your heart or your brain, because your heart and brain are too sensitive to the intense hand-chi energy. But you can energize your eyes, nose, mouth, jaw, ears, neck, throat, etc. Actually, you can put hand-chi into any area of your body that you want to, except for your heart, brain, or perhaps some injured, oversensitive area.

Whenever a part of my body gets "struck" or "injured", for decades now I've energized my palms and put them both (stacked: one hand on the other) on top of that "struck" or "injured" area, to promote healing, from all the intensely energizing hand chi. You can experiment with this, too, to see if this also will work for you (it should).

Anyway, try all this. It's really quite powerful! In fact, it's like Reiki (giving chi, from a raised hand, at a distance), but even more powerful, because the energy is given so close up, right to the body.

When this energy tool is used on others, it's called "healing hands".

Energy Tool

#18. Chi Gong (Chinese Yoga)

Chi Gong (or Chinese yoga) is a 6,000-year-old practice of increasing energy in your body. Chi Gong can powerfully heal you, energize you thoroughly, and transform your whole life!

The very best book on Chi Gong seems to be Suzanne B. Friedman's book, "Heal Yourself With Qigong" (Qigong is just a different way to spell Chi Gong). Get this book, read it, and experimentally try the techniques, if you want lots more energy!

Other books and DVDs on Chi Gong exist, but what is truly needed here is a book written by a Westerner who thoroughly understands Chi Gong, so that it can all be clearly explained to other Westerners in a way that "demystifies" Chi Gong. Suzanne Friedmen does exactly this, which is why it's perhaps the very best book!

Enough said, here. Buy it, and do it, to energize yourself abundantly!

Energy Tool

#19. Chi-Nei-Tsang

The ability of our stomach and gut, to digest food and give us energy, is extremely important! Obviously!

Well, there is an ancient Chinese technique (6,000 years old) of very gently massaging most of the digestive organs (from below the bottom rib to just above the pelvic area). You periodically (and very gently) massage the stomach, pancreas, small intestine, upper large intestine, liver, gallbladder, kidneys, and bladder (etc.). This tonifies all these digestive organs with chi-energy, so that you can better digest your food. And, the more you gently massage them all, the healthier they become, so that food digestion and absorption become better and better! Is it clear how this all works?

This is especially good for middle-aged or older people with digestive problems, including "leaky bowel syndrome".

"Fingertip shiatsu" is the massage technique for doing this. Gently place your fingertips on your gut area, and make little circular massage motions, as you gently press in. You'll be able to feel the right amount of gentle pressure to use. Experiment over the whole gut area with this "fingertip shiatsu" technique, as you slowly improve on it, day by day. Or, have your spouse gently try it on you, as they slowly learn it.

You might try a search on the internet, on "Chi Nei Tsang".

A good book on this is Mantak Chia's "Chi Nei Tsang", available on the internet. Chinese medicine practitioners, who do acupuncture, or prescribe Chinese herbs, may be able to refer you to someone who actually does Chi Nei Tsang professionally for perhaps $75? I, myself, after reading the above book, went to a professional Chi Nei Tsang practitioner for one time only.

I carefully observed what was done to my gut, asked many questions, and then felt that I knew enough to start gently doing Chi Nei Tsang on myself. You could try this too, because it's best to learn how to do it on yourself—for free—and frequently!

Do this on an empty stomach! Go slow! Back off if you encounter any pain, after which you should do it less and even more gently. Try it!

Energy Tool

#20. Chinese Dietary Therapy

(This is not about eating Chinese food in Chinese restaurants!)

The very powerful and healing Chinese Medical System (6,000 years old!) has rated thousands of herbs, as to their healing properties. But also, it has rated many ordinarily-eaten foods, as to the healing properties of these foods!

Chinese Dietary Therapy involves eating those foods that most heal you, according to your present physical condition.

There is available on the internet a book entitled "Prince Wen Hui's Cook; Chinese Dietary Therapy", by Bob Flaws and Honora Wolf (copyright 1983). This very valuable book rates the healing value of hundreds of ordinarily-eaten foods.

A dietary plan for fatigued, exhausted, run-down people is on page 39, and includes all the 37 most tonifying, energizing foods there are, including oats, cooked squash, cooked sweet potatoes, and cooked yams (as the 4 very best of them). Recommended foods and dietary plans for other less-than-healthy conditions are given, too.

Anyone who would like to recover their health quickly, and to have lots more energy derived from dietary sources, would be well-advised to get this book and apply it, by fixing and eating the recommended healing foods here!

Energy Tool

#21. Chinese Tonic Pills

In the herbology branch of Chinese Medicine (6,000 years old) there are numerous herbs that "tonify" your body, and give you energy. Formulas of several herbs have been created, to energize your body in the most efficient way possible! A company in Holland converts these tonic herbs into pill-capsules, and sells them (relatively inexpensively) through this organization: "Institute For Traditional Medicine", 2017 S.E. Hawthorne, Portland, Oregon 97217 [telephone numbers: (800) 544-7504 and (503) 233-4907].

Their "Bu Zhong Yi Qi Wan" (ginseng & astragalus formula) is very energizing and tonifying to take! Also, their "Liu Wei Di Huang Wan" (rehmannia six formula) is quite energizing and tonifying to the body, too! (The cost of both is relatively low.)

I highly recommend ordering these 2 formulas, to take daily, if you want to greatly increase your energy!

Also, a local health food store sells a similarly-effective product called "Supreme Blend Chi Tonic" (a daily tonic for energy & vitality, that's energetically activating). This can be ordered online at Medicinal-Foods.com (if your local health food store doesn't carry it).

Energy Tool

#22. Chiropractic-Towel-Under-Spine Technique

Once my girlfriend took me to an incredible "Super Stretching Class" taught by an excellent professional woman chiropractor. After doing several slightly complicated stretches (directed by this woman in her class) my body felt absolutely amazing. In fact, my body felt better than ever before (or since) in my life!

Normally, in every class I've ever taken, I'm busy taking very rapid notes, recording everything as precisely as I can. And, this is normally what I would have done here. But since I was sort of my girlfriend's "guest" at the class, my habitual rapid note-taking might have seemed too "weird ", both to her and all the others there.

Thus, all the ultra-wonderful stretches were lost to me, except for this #1 technique, which was repeated in every class (as all the other taught stretches kept varying).

Directions for Chiropractic-Towel-Under-Spine Technique (Chiropractic Yoga?):

1. Roll up a small towel and place it in the middle of a large rug. The rolled-up towel should then look like a cylinder, that's soft and yielding.

2. Lie down on the rug (on your back) so that your head is above the rolled-up towel, your neck is directly over the towel, and the rest of your body is below the rolled-up towel. Your legs are also very bent so that your knees are pointed upward, toward the ceiling.

3. Now, very slowly (and gently and carefully) move your body up over the towel, using your arms and legs to do this.

4. Very gradually, move every one of your back's vertebrae up and over the rolled-up towel (that's serving as a very soft, yielding cylinder, on the rug).

5. You've started with a small towel, so that the raising and lowering of each vertebrae (up, over, and down around the towel) will be as easily done as possible, in your first experience, here. Later, you can use a bigger or thicker towel, for greater effect, if you want (in the future).

6. As you gently, slowly, and carefully lift each of your back's vertebrae up and over the rolled-up-cylindrical-soft-towel, you'll eventually get to your last (tailbone) vertebrae. After doing this last one, reverse directions, and very gradually go back to where you started.

7. After you've done all this stretching of your back's vertebrae,

your back will feel utterly amazing and super-stretched! In fact, after doing all this "vertebrae-over-the-towel" technique, you may feel better emotionally, and be more energy-filled, than ever!

Note. If your back is in any way fragile or very old, be quite careful with this technique. Perhaps you can share all this with a licensed chiropractor, and do it carefully (for the first time) under their professional supervision?

Anyway, for a bursting-with-vitality, limbered-up, relaxed healthy spine that feels almost "super-human", this is the very best technique to use!

Energy Tool

#23. Circadian Rhythms

Our energy/vitality level seems to vary throughout the day! Sometimes we're high energy, sometimes medium energy, and sometimes low energy (in a slump).

Almost everyone has heard of "morning people" (high energy in the morning), or night people (high energy at night). There are also "afternoon people" and "swing-shift people" (high energy from 4 PM to midnight).

The biological reason why our energy varies (over a 24-hour period) is that various organs in our body are undergoing a multitude of physiological processes, regularly at a certain hour, every day! As far as I know, we're pretty much stuck with our highly individual circadian rhythms, precisely because they're linked to these bodily processes (in multiple organs) in us.

Well, we can do something about these circadian rhythms, but we first need to know their pattern! In fact, if you even had a graph of them, you could really use this graph to your advantage, in best utilizing your energy throughout every day.

I once made a graph of my circadian rhythms that I created by intuitively (and emotionally) tuning into the amount of physical energy I had, at every specific hour of every day. Over time, I verified the accuracy of my estimations of the "degree of energeticness" during every specific hour of the day. Eventually, I was amazed at how precise this "energy graph" was!

I have worked with my specific graph for decades now, in deciding when to sleep, to nap, to meditate, to be more active physically, and to be most active mentally. For, obviously, my best work occurs when I have the best and the most energy. Right?

Conclusion. Create your very own "circadian energy graph", fine-tune it, and experimentally work with it. It's utterly invaluable in managing your energy, best. Once you have your own very personal energy rhythms graph, you'll wonder how you ever got through your day without it!

So, first, create a "rough draft" of your energy graph, then fine-tune it and correct it, as you experience your energy-level shifts at different times of the day. Then, learn to work with your energy graph, slowly but surely, over time. Best of luck to you, here!

Energy Tool

#24. Colloidal Silver (For COVID-19 Help)

Colloidal silver used to be the doctors' and mainstream medicine's #1 antibiotic, from about 1880 to 1950. There actually were a few dozen antibiotics, containing trillions of microscopic particles of silver (very deadly to all germs) during this 70-year period.

Colloidal silver (and other similar antibiotics containing microscopic silver particles) is superior to penicillin, because colloidal silver kills viruses too, whereas penicillin (and many other "modern" antibiotics) kills only bacteria but not viruses.

There are some good, informative books on the internet that explain practically everything about colloidal silver. It's very important to read them thoroughly, in order to best, and knowledgeably, use this incredible wonder-antibiotic, colloidal silver! I recommend John Hill's "Colloidal Silver" and Warren Jefferson's "Colloidal Silver Today".

It's shocking that health practitioners haven't come forward in informing the American public as to how effective colloidal silver is, in treating all viruses (including the COVID-19 virus).

Now, it seems to be the case that antibiotics aren't that good to take if you're healthy, because antibiotics kill the helpful probiotic bacteria (in your gut) that assist digestion, etc. But, if you're quite sick, with a bacteria or virus (that needs to be immediately destroyed) then taking colloidal silver is very appropriate, especially if it's a life-threatening virus, like COVID-19.

Anyway, educate yourself on colloidal silver via internet books, read thoroughly. You'll really be glad you did and then have colloidal silver as a tool to stop germs from wrecking your energy!

P.S. Colloidal silver never turned anyone's skin gray. This is a myth and outright lie, to discredit this wonderful antibiotic and antiviral. Both books above explain all this thoroughly.

P.P.S. Colloidal silver can perhaps be combined with vitamin C injections, to eradicate viruses. See Energy Tool #95.

Energy Tool

#25. Color Therapy Glasses (Green)

On the internet, you can find tinted glasses (non-prescription) for sale, called "color therapy glasses". These glasses are in over a dozen colors, and each tinted color tends to put you in a different mood, psychologically!

Green color therapy glasses tend to make you feel like you're in a forest of greenery, which relaxes and soothes you (like in meditating). In fact, these green-tinted glasses are perfect for those who aren't into meditating. Simply put on the green specs, instead, to soothe your mind and emotions!

Because green color therapy glasses relax you, soothe you, and make you happier, they're a great break from the stress of a job. They're almost like a "semi-nap"! Then, when you take them off, afterward, you're refreshed and have more energy to continue to work!

You can experiment with the other colors (besides green), too. Red color therapy glasses supposedly (in the instructions) energize you more. But I found this was true for only a 5 or 10 minute "burst of energy", followed by greater exhaustion. Therefore, I'd recommend using the green glasses for rest, followed by more energy later!

Incidentally, gold or amber (not yellow) color therapy glasses make you happier, stopping depression. Of course, gold and amber glasses only temporarily "repress" the depression, as aromatherapies do. But still, a more joyful mood for 5 minutes can give you the positive energy to get going on a new project or chore. Try it!

Energy Tool

#26. Color, Wear Your Favorite –

There's a reason why you have a favorite color. It's because that color extremely resonates with your personality! Thus, this favorite color actually gives energy to your personality and charges it up. Yes!

Now obviously, to dress completely in your favorite color (in public) would appear weird, to others. When do we ever see someone dressed in all red, all orange, all yellow, all green, all blue, or all purple? Not often! So, wear as much of your favorite color as you "stylishly" can, but blend in a few other colors to that to (sort of) match it. Then you'll be energized by wearing as much of your favorite color as you possibly can, when you're in public.

But what about in private? Isn't that a totally different matter? When you're alone, and away from any spying or prying eyes, then (yes!) try dressing totally in your favorite color. Then, alone and by yourself, you can be completely charged up. Try it!

Once alone and dressed totally in your favorite color, you should be so energized and charged up that you'll have the passion, vitality, and willpower to do many more things that you couldn't quite do before! So, make use of this extra power and energy to accomplish (alone) some pretty extraordinary things. In fact, accomplish things you may never have even thought possible! (Isn't this almost a bit like Clark Kent changing his outfit to turn into Superman? Or Diana Prince changing her outfit to turn into Wonder Woman?)

Good luck!

P.S. If you have two favorite colors, try alternating them. Or, even blending them! Also, you might discover that one color helps you to best do mental work, another color helps you to best do physical work, and two other colors help you to do emotional work and intuitive work. Enjoyably try experimenting, here!

Energy Tool

#27. Crying Out Woes, To Re-Energize

Babies and little children automatically cry out their woes. Crying is a natural, instinctive way to release so-called "negative" emotions. After a good cry, we feel we've released a lot of these "negative" emotions, and we feel much better. Also, it takes energy to repress all our "negative" emotions, so that when these "negative" emotions are cried out, we no longer have to waste energy repressing them. Thus, a good cry-out eventually results in more (and more positive) energy!

Enter Society, with all its shame and ridiculing of crying. This very much represses the crying ability in most of us. Even today, when crying is heard behind a closed door, the one who hears us is often disgusted and thinks we're being "childish". (Especially for men, where there's practically a taboo against crying.)

"Ninja Crying" is the solution, here. We greatly need to use this crying-it-out tool, but it must be done secretly, in a ninja-like way, to avoid "shameful" discovery by others.

Here are some Ninja Crying methods, to "cry-on-the-sly":

1. Cry in the shower, with the water running hard. If you don't "wail" too loud, the sound of the shower water should mask the sound of your crying. Crying moderately as the bathtub fills loudly can mask the sound of crying, too.

2. Crying for just 3 to 5 seconds as the toilet flushes works, for a brief and quick "release of grief".

3. Crying in your car, when parked in a deserted, isolated spot at night, works. But don't get mugged out there, in that ultra-deserted spot.

4. Semi-crying while walking around in the rain can work. Compose your face back to "normal" whenever someone walks closely by you.

5. Cry behind a COVID-19 face mask, if you can be well away from others so that you won't be heard.

6. Cry under the covers of your bed. This greatly mutes the noise.

7. Relax your vocal chords so much, when crying, that only slight air-hiss sounds are heard. Do this when crying at home, or in the private toilet stall, at work.

8. Go to a cemetery (wearing black?) Pick a random grave, and sob over it! This works with pet cemeteries, too. You might even meet someone special, as when "Harold" met "Maude".

9. Be creative, and find your own "Ninja Crying" methods that work especially for you. Be really "out there" with this. (Start a

"Crying Club"? Even one that holds fake funerals in graveyards? Ha, ha. Go for it!)

Conclusion. Crying is such a powerful, natural remedy for releasing "negativity" (and thus feeling more energy) that you really should give it a go with some effective ways to "ninja-cry-on-the-sly". Right? Don't you owe it to yourself, to provide for yourself, this ultimate remedy to transformatively release the inner despair and sadness of your soul?

P.S. If you're a man reading this, then "ninja-crying-on-the-sly" won't make you any less of a tough-macho soldier, or take away your "ticket to the men's-club". No one will know, you'll feel better and more energized, and with all this added energy you'll be an even greater tough warrior-soldier, all lean-and-mean. Right? Think about it!

P.P.S. Remember what Mark Twain once quipped: "90% of all people need to cry it out, and the other 10%-in-denial (who say they don't need to) are liars!"

Energy Tool

#28. Dance Out Stressful Emotions

The stressful emotions of depression, fear, anxiety, anger, etc., all reduce our goal of using our energy to create a happier and more successful life. Well then, dance them out! By dancing out stressful emotions, they'll be released or reduced, so that you can energetically get your life back on track!

Gabrielle Roth's book "Sweat Your Prayers" is an utterly excellent book on the methodology of dancing out any troubling emotions you're having. Check it out!

The American Indians had a war dance, a hunting dance, a rain dance, and a sun dance, etc. Well, you can have an anger-out dance, a depression-stop dance, and a fear-begone dance. Right? Perhaps these three dances could also be called a swearing-yelling-dance, a crying-sobbing-dance, and a shaking-trembling-dance, depending on your own personal, unique way of dancing these dances. Incidentally, Rajneesh (or Osho) created many dances/meditations along this line. Look them up, in his books and DVDs.

Anyway, be creative here, and create the dance forms that you personally need, to dance out the unpleasant emotions that are troubling you. Afterward, when these stressful emotions are released or reduced, you'll once again have the energy to resume creating a happy and successful life!

Energy Tool

#29. Deep Breathing For More Oxygen

Most of us breathe rather shallowly, due to outer (and inner) stress. This results in insufficient oxygen intake. Yet, oxygen is an extremely important ingredient in our cellular chemical reactions that produce energy.

It's almost as if Einstein's famous formula could be instead: $E = O \cdot c^2$, where the "O" is oxygen!

The solution to this is called "Full Breathing". Try to:

(1) relax your lungs as much as possible as you breathe, and

(2) allow your diaphragm (just below your lungs) to inflate first, before your lungs do;

(3) keep inhaling until your lungs are a bit more full (than you typically breathe), then

(4) exhale, to start over again.

Do this "Full Breathing" technique ten times, then stop and resume your typical pattern of breathing again. (Don't do it more than ten times at first, until you get more used to it. Also, it's pretty important to get books on deeper breathing techniques, and learn a lot more about all this, if you want to get more advanced beyond this simple beginner's technique.)

You should feel more energy from these ten full breaths! Also, it often helps you to feel calmer and more grounded, too.

Do this "Full Breathing" technique whenever you need an energy boost, but probably not more than three times per day (until you've educated yourself, by books or DVDs on all the possible effects and side effects of doing this more).

Isn't it a bit fun to just "breathe in" more energy, for free, whenever you want to? It works! (As long as you don't overdo it, at first.)

P.S. This deeper breathing could lead to some yawning (Energy Tool #99). If so, let yourself start "yawning away"!

P.P.S. A friend of mine told me of an alternative breathing technique, for beginners:

(1) Breathe in, in 3 stages, filling up your lungs about 1/3 each time. In other words, breathe in 1/3, breathe in 1/3, breathe in 1/3.

(2) Then exhale normally.

(3) Then breathe in normally.

(4) Then breathe out 1/3, breathe out 1/3, breathe out 1/3.

(5) Then repeat (1).

(6) Then repeat (4).

(7) Then repeat this whole sequence two more times, and stop! Try it, and see how much more energized it makes you feel.

Energy Tool

#30. Diet Greatly Helps Your Energy!

Eat sensibly, with foods and drinks that nourish your body! Avoid junk foods that just make any exhaustion worse. Also, avoid sweets, which at first give you a quick "sugar rush", but then lead to severe drops in blood sugar levels, later. A lower blood sugar level will make it much harder to continue to stay energized.

Also, try not to overeat. Fill up with more fruits and vegetables. Try having small meals, but more frequently. Eat more protein, healthy fats (coconut oil, organic butter, fish), and non-starchy vegetables to give you more energy that lasts! Eat a well-balanced diet, to give your body the 100 nutrients it needs every day. Eating eggs, yogurt, cheese, fish, and beans, in your meals and snacks, provides essential amino acids, probiotics, and healthy fats that will provide the energy and healthiness you need, to offset fatigue.

Organic foods in your diet usually give you much more nutrition and fewer toxins, than non-organic foods, and are especially needed by your body. Focus on eating the very healthiest, now, to maximize your body's energy through nutrition!

Energy Tool

#31. Dual Brain Psychology

Fredric Schiffer, M.D., who was a successful surgeon, psychiatrist, and Harvard lecturer, wrote an outstanding book entitled "Of Two Minds", on Dual Brain Psychology. In a clear and extremely intelligent way, with abundant evidence cited and top-quality writing skills, Dr. Schiffer proves conclusively that the two hemispheres of our brain are actually two different personalities that often alternate in our behavior and in our life!

One of our personality-hemispheres is usually reasonably healthy, stable, down-to-earth, grown-up, and has plenty of common sense, Dr. Schiffer found. But our other personality-hemisphere is often very adolescent-like or even kid-like, is full of anger, depression, fear, and angst; is strongly affected by all our unhealed traumas from the past, and often is addicted to harmful things. It acts quite immaturely and capriciously more often than not! (This immature hemisphere can be either the left brain hemisphere or the right brain hemisphere, it turns out.)

Do you see what this means? It explains our "inner war", mixed feelings, lack of unity, and inner sabotaging that we often feel inside ourselves. It sheds light on why we often genuinely want to do (or say) one thing, but end up doing (or saying) another!

The way to begin to heal this inner Dual Brain turmoil is for the more mature hemispheric self to understand, befriend, nurture, counsel, and attempt to slowly heal the more immature hemispheric self. Only in this way can the two hemispheric selves begin to work as a team-of-two, instead of as adversaries, continually thwarting and sabotaging the other hemispheric personality's goals! But note that all this is definitely not "inner child work", Dr. Schiffer emphatically states, because both hemispheric personalities are well-established adults living and functioning in the world (even though one of these adults behaves rather un-adultlike, on occasion).

Because of the astounding factual truth of what you've just read, and absolutely need to confirm this by reading Dr. Schiffer's book "Of Two Minds", this is the most important of all these 101 energy tools! For, how can your "mature hemispheric you" successfully energize yourself with these 101 tools for long, when your "immature hemispheric you" will just turn around and sabotage and wreck any ongoing program of bodily energization?

Incidentally, your "immature/adolescent-like or kid-like hemispheric you" will also sabotage or compromise your career, financial stability, marriage, relationships, interactions with your children and friends, health, hobbies, and personal and spiritual growth programs, too! No wonder your personal history is so "checkered" with so many disturbing signs of inner disunity!

It's extremely important that I alert you to the inner discord between your two hemispheric personality selves (due to their not working successfully as a team-of-two). For, only by reading Dr. Schiffer's excellent and amazing explanatory book (and beginning an inner program of your mature-self befriending and starting to heal your immature-self), can any real and lasting progress in your life's goals finally be made!

Does all this make sense? How can a "house divided" progress onward in just about anything? Right?

So, in conclusion, the absolute greatest energy and happiness tool you can ever do, is to read Dr. Schiffer's "Of Two Minds". (Incidentally, I've read and reread this incredible book five times, and it's completely changed the course of my life. In fact, this book you're now holding wouldn't have been written without my having followed Dr. Schiffer's inner-befriending-and-healing-program because my immature-hemisphere was absolutely refusing to finish writing this book!)

To truly succeed in filling your life with great energy and happiness, you really need to read Dr. Schiffer's book "Of Two Minds". Please do it! Please don't ignore this wise advice, here! Okay?

Energy Tool

#32. $E = m \cdot c^2$, Not $E = m \cdot J^2$

It might be surprising to see Einstein's famous formula here, but actually, it's extremely appropriate! See, plants need quality matter (soil minerals, pure water, CO_2 molecules, and sunlight's photon particles) to produce abundant energy through photosynthesis. Likewise, animals need quality matter (healthy food, required vitamins and minerals, pure water, and oxygen molecules) to produce abundant energy through digestion.

In other words, quality matter is supremely important in creating quality-abundant energy! But it's exactly this that numerous people just aren't "getting" when they eat junk food, drink impure water, breathe polluted air, don't recharge their body's digestive system with sufficient sleep, and pollute their body with alcohol, cigarettes, drugs, and all the 450-or-so environmental toxins in non-organic food.

How can abundant energy be produced in a body that's stuffed with so much "junk-garbage" that it's practically turned into a semi-cesspool? The abundant-energy producing formula is *not*:

$E = m \cdot J^2$ (where "J" is Junk-garbage).

Get it? Our bodies, like the bodies of all animals in nature, are natural and nature-based. Do we see animals in nature stuffing their natural bodies with junky garbage? And, if they did, how much energy would they have to outrun predators and survive in the jungle's rather harsh habitat? Do you get the point, here?

Almost all the energy tools in this book encourage the ingesting of "good stuff" for energy and avoiding the "bad stuff" that wrecks and reduces energy. So, start applying $E = m \cdot c^2$, instead of $E = m \cdot J^2$, then begin dramatically increasing your energy, starting today!

Energy Tool

#33. Ear Acupressure Massage

An excellent method to pull yourself out of low energy and depression is to thoroughly massage your ears! I know this sounds rather odd, but your ears contain dozens of acupressure points that, when pressed, give you energy and more happiness!

There used to be available on the internet, little plastic "model ears" for sale, marked with about 50 to 100 acupuncture points. But rather than memorizing any points from these ear models (or from internet ear charts that you can find) simply press "the heck" all over your ears, thoroughly. Do the outside-the-ear points, inside-the-ear points, and even gently rub up and down in the back—and in front—of your ears. Press every bit of your ear's surface area, and also around your ears (including pinching gently your ear lobes).

It helps greatly to position your thumbs inside your ears, and position your index and middle fingers (opposite your thumbs) on the outside of your ears. Then, just pinch your thumbs and index/middle fingers together. Do this again and again, over the entire surface area of your ears, simultaneously getting both the inner and outer points at the same time. Do both ears at once, this way!

Obviously, when you press the most central ear points (in your ear canal's opening) it's important to have clean, washed fingers, to avoid giving yourself an ear infection (from the germs on dirty fingertips).

You'll find that this ear acupressure massage tool is an excellent, fast way to both level up your mood, and increase your energy.

Energy Tool

#34. Earth Power Spots & Feng Shui

There are certain spots on the earth that can greatly empower you! Often they are in the mountains, or on a hill. They can be in a forest, or near a huge tree, or on a lake or beach. You can even create your own power spot by designing a beautiful backyard garden, and filling it with special power objects, and using "power-spot-creating technologies".

Feng shui (the ancient Chinese art of empowering your health and success by the harmonious arrangement of objects in your home) can be employed here too, to great effect.

Interior decorating, using common sense and your favorite color combinations, works well also.

Basically, the idea here is to empower your: home, yard, car, clothes, workplace, and every environment around you (under your control) to serve more as a battery that recharges and energizes you!

Or, alternatively, you can create or visit (frequently) the authentic earth-power-spots in your vicinity.

So, go for it!

Energy Tool

#35. Enema Hose In Shower

Regularly cleaning out the very end of your large intestine will give you more energy! This is because very often fecal matter gets backed up in the large intestine, and with either "leaky bowel syndrome", or "semi-leaky bowel syndrome", the toxins and bacteria in this fecal matter can partially end up right back in your bloodstream, greatly reducing your energy.

The solution to this is to buy (on the internet) a metal (or plastic) enema hose that conveniently hooks up to your shower spout. It gives you easy enemas that take just a few seconds. A quick click at the top of the enema hose switches the water to the hose, and another quick click switches the water back to the shower spout. Only a very short (2- or 3-second) burst of water up inside, then a quick expelling, will quickly get rid of any fecal re-absorption problems, here.

People who've tried this all report they instantly felt quite a bit more energy, when they quickly cleaned themselves out with the shower's enema hose.

Consider trying this energy tool. It really works, and it's so quick and effective!

Energy Tool

#36. Ester-C (For COVID Help)

There is a powerful form of vitamin C that's buffered (with either calcium or magnesium). By being buffered like this, huge amounts of vitamin C can enter your stomach without upsetting it, since the calcium or magnesium neutralizes the acidity of the (ascorbic acid) vitamin C.

Colds and flu, plus viral and bacterial diseases can be "blasted away" with megadoses of Ester-C, since vitamin C is so extremely effective in killing off germs (in your bloodstream) fast!

Ester-C works very effectively in lessening the symptoms of COVID-19 too (and I'm surprised it hasn't been mentioned more in the press). Unfortunately, there is often a side effect of taking a lot of Ester-C, and it's diarrhea. Be sure you're near a bathroom when taking a lot of Ester-C, because you may soon end up running there.

Injections of vitamin C into the blood are even more effective against germs and diseases, but either a medical practitioner or special skill might be needed here, to safely administer these injections. Adelle Davis, in her book "Let's Eat Right To Keep Fit" (page 131 line 31 and page 132 lines 1, 8, 9, 20, 24, and 34, and page 133 line 41) mentions these very powerful injections of vitamin C into the blood (done by doctors, and in traditional hospitals, in the 1950s); she tells how incredibly effective injections of vitamin C are against numerous diseases, so much so, that vitamin C is practically a "miracle drug"!

Colloidal silver, in very high concentrations, is also quite effective in killing germs (including COVID-19). (See Energy Tool #24.) Colloidal silver was extensively used by medical doctors, and in traditional hospitals, from 1880 to about 1950.

To sum up, start using these very powerful vitamin C techniques to fight diseases, and restore your energy!

Energy Tool

#37. Favorite (Healthy) Meal To Fix

Almost nothing empowers you as much as fixing and eating your favorite healthy meal. What is it that you really enjoy eating (that's healthy) more than anything else? Well then, fix it and eat it!

If your favorite (of all meals) can only be experienced at a certain restaurant, then go there fairly often (if it's not too expensive). And, if fixing your favorite meal requires some training or expertise, then make the effort to acquire those skills, for it will be well worth it! Learn by computer, or through a friend with cooking skills, or even the right class.

We all have our favorite-favorite meal (although this can change, as the years go by). So, treat yourself to it! Do it as often as you can (without tiring yourself of it, by overdose).

By pleasuring and rewarding yourself often (with your favorite meal) and super-nurturing yourself in this way, your inner happiness and contentment will energize and motivate you to do the work necessary to create the best possible life for yourself!

Energy Tool

#38. Five-Minute Massage Of 30 Muscles

Almost everyone loves a massage. Unfortunately, they're expensive and time-consuming. And it's a "hassle" to do it to yourself. But this is a technique that gets around all this! Because, you'll only be spending 5 minutes on self-massage, yet get 30 muscles! And even though this averages only 10 seconds per muscle, it's well worth it. After all, each muscle getting massaged (for only 10 seconds) is better than nothing at all!

Here are your 30 muscles/body parts to massage:

1. Right hand and fingers
2. Right forearm and elbow
3. Right upper arm
4. Right shoulder
5. Left hand and fingers
6. Left forearm and elbow
7. Left upper arm
8. Left shoulder
9. Right foot
10. Right lower leg and ankle
11. Right upper leg and knee
12. Right buttock (reaching behind, with fist)
13. Left foot
14. Left lower leg and ankle
15. Left upper leg and knee
16. Left buttock (reaching behind, with fist)
17. Right side (from hip joint to armpit)
18. Left side (from hip joint to armpit)
19. Stomach (gently)
20. Chest and pectorals
21. Trapezius muscle (between neck and shoulders)
22. Neck
23. Jaw
24. Ears
25. Forehead
26. Scalp (called Indian Head Massage)

27. Right lower back (reaching your knuckles up behind you)

28. Left lower back (reaching your knuckles up behind you)

29. Upper back (using a massage stick or tool, like my Back Roller Massager (Energy tool #9) or a "lomilomi stick", or a Theracane (ordered on the internet).

30. Any remaining area that possibly got left out on this list, that needs attention.

Definitely massage all these areas in any order that you want. You could try counting off the ten seconds—from 1 to 10—as you massage each area.

So, now you have it! Rapidly, and as skillfully as you can, "blitz-massage", for 10 seconds, each of these 30 body areas, to afterward feel utterly "super", and re-energized once again!

Repeated practice of this will make you better and better, over time!

If you have 10 minutes (instead of just 5) for self-massage, count from 1 to 20 (seconds) for each area that you're massaging.

You could try following this Blitz-Massage with Energy Tool #52: Meditation (soothing and relaxing). This greatly helps you to recover your equilibrium, afterward!

Treat yourself to this 5-minute (or 10-minute) massage as often as you want. At work, you'll probably have to do it while hidden from sight, in a restroom stall, or in your car (out in the parking lot).

Energy Tool

#39. Foods That Are Very Nutritional To Eat

There are four incredibly nutritional foods that need to be included in your diet as often as possible. These are:

1. oats (organic is best),
2. yams and sweet potatoes (organic is best),
3. zucchini and squash (organic is best),
4. Dave's Killer Bread (organic bread with 21 whole grains and seeds).

All four of these are amazingly nourishing, and especially help to give you energy if you're run down, depleted in energy, fatigued, or exhausted!

Try them and see!

Obviously, 1., 2., and 3. need to be cooked slowly at low heat, in order to preserve the nutrients in them.

Energy Tool

#40. Ginseng

Ginseng often gives you more energy. Nibbling on a ginseng root can contribute to energizing you more. Chewing 1-2 grams off the end of a root delivers a standard daily dose. Ginseng can be subtle, but it tonifies, energizes, and increases alertness. A standardized extract of 4% to 7% ginsenosides seems to give the best results and benefits.

Ginseng increases physical endurance and stamina.

With ginseng powder, try adding a teaspoon to your morning meal, to help boost your physical energy.

Ginseng needs to be taken for two weeks, then not taken for two weeks! Taking ginseng with ginger helps a lot, too. With this schedule of "two weeks on and two weeks off" ginseng, you avoid any possible "ginseng overdose" side effects.

Take ginseng before noon, or its energizing properties may interfere with your sleep that night (if taken after noon).

Ginseng, for several reasons, can be an excellent help in adding energy to your physical body!

Energy Tool

#41. Hands Clasp

When energy, or life force, or "chi" is circulating around your body, some of it gradually drains out from your hands and feet. By clasping your hands together, any energy that would have drained out of your right hand is reabsorbed into your left hand and goes up your left arm. Also, any energy that would have drained out of your left hand, is reabsorbed into your right hand and goes up your right arm. So, you tend to keep your energy from this technique, and not have it drain out!

Thus, by putting your hands together in several different clasping or "hand-holding" positions, you keep more of your energy circulating in your body, instead of having it drain out. You can also do this by clasping the right wrist or forearm with your left hand, or by clasping the left wrist or forearm with the right hand (or both). Crossing your arms is an effective "clasp" that stops energy draining from the hands and arms, too. Placing both palms over your "belly button" helps greatly, also (with one palm on top of the other palm). Cupping your elbows with opposite palms can also work.

The feet can help in this energy-saving, too, by being put together, or crossed at the ankles (etc.). Experiment!

Several "hatha yoga" sitting positions are designed to maintain your energy, by stopping any draining-of-the-energy from either hands or feet. Analytical thinking seems to be helped by this clasping, too, especially if one (or both) hands clasps the head in some way!

Putting one or both hands in your pockets, or even hugging yourself, helps, too.

Doing this clasping in the evening, or late at night, especially helps you to maintain your energy, until bedtime.

Try experimenting with different varieties of all this, to find your most favorite hand and feet clasps or positionings that help you to avoid losing your energy!

Energy Tool

#42. Hatha Yoga

Over the years, I have had many friends who absolutely raved about how good they felt physically, by doing Hatha Yoga daily. When I was 19, I learned the basic 10 or so asanas (yoga postures) and did them all daily, for a while. I still remember many of their Indian names: the plow, locust, cobra, twist, shoulderstand, headstand, full lotus, half lotus, lion, "dead pose", etc.

Much later, I even attended a few yoga classes and felt great (physically) afterward.

Do a search on the internet for the best modern books and/or DVDs on Hatha Yoga, paying special attention to the customer's reviews. Are these customers reporting they're feeling "really great" after their Hatha Yoga session? If so, then buy this book or DVD!

Once a friend told me that the book "Light On Yoga" was really excellent.

If you have the discipline to follow a brief and effective Hatha Yoga routine daily, your body will start feeling wonderful, and full of energy, fast. Try it!

Energy Tool

#43. Hot Baths

Hot baths are invigorating, especially when things are added to the water, like salts and aromatherapies, etc. Toxins are sweated out, and negative emotional energies in you are sort of "washed away". Also, you become more relaxed, which helps you to re-energize.

Many women already know all this about baths, and much more! If you're a man, go ask a woman, and she'll tell you all about this. Also, the internet will give you many valuable tips, here.

So, try hot baths. They work!

Energy Tool

#44. HSO Probiotics

There is a super form of probiotics called HSOs. It stands for "Homeostatic Soil Organisms". (Look it up on the internet.) HSOs are very powerful in killing off the "bad guys" in your digestive tract, and greatly increasing your absorbability of food.

Jordan Rubin's book "Restoring Your Digestive Health" (available on the internet) thoroughly describes the incredibleness of HSOs, in greatly improving your health and energy! The "Garden of Life" brand "Primal Defense" (HSO Probiotics Formula-Helps Maintain Digestive Health!) is a very good one to buy. It can be ordered at www.gardenoflife.com.

Try it, and see your energy increase dramatically!

Energy Tool

#45. Indian Head Massage

In the West, this is simply called "scalp massage", and is skillfully done with the fingertips. The object is to manipulate the skin of the scalp (and not just rub the hair around).

In the East, especially in India, it's called Indian Head Massage because it's thousands of years old, and is the favorite type of massage in India. Children in India are often given a daily head massage until they're four years old, and after that twice weekly.

Two excellent books on this are "Mind-Blowing Head Massage", by Francesca Rinaldi, and "The Art of Indian Head Massage", by Mary Atkinson. Besides the entire head and scalp, the face, neck, shoulders, upper back, and upper arms can be included too. It's an excellent therapy for relieving the stress of modern living, giving relaxation, peace of mind, and harmony of body and soul.

So, reach your hands up to your head, scalp, neck, and shoulders often, to treat yourself to an energizing Indian Head Massage whenever you feel the need for it. Try it!

P.S. Using the Roller Massager (Energy Tool #74) on your head, is a quick, easy, and very effective way to do Indian Head Massage, too. Try this especially, also!

Energy Tool

#46. Isometrics

Isometrics have been around for over 50 years. (You may have heard of them.) Basically, isometric exercise is pushing a muscle against resistance, without moving your body much. For example, extend your forearms (only) out in front of you, with hands clasped. Put your left hand on the top, and your right hand on the bottom. Your upper arms are relaxed at your sides, but your elbows are bent 90 degrees, so it's only your forearms extended out. Now, muscularly push down with your (on top) left forearm, as (simultaneously) you push up with your right forearm (on bottom). Since your two hands are clasped together, this opposite pushing with the two forearms usually results in little movement (only some quivering). This is because the left and right forearm muscles are sort of canceling each other out. Right? Get the principle here?

Thus, both forearm muscles are pushing hard, and are strongly exercising, yet there's almost no movement with your clasped hands.

By exercising many of your muscles in this way, you'll build muscle mass gradually, which will then slowly give you more energy! You'll also be fitter and in shape.

There are several books and DVDs on isometrics (on the internet) that you can buy. Try setting up your own personal daily isometric program!

Isometric exercise is ideal for people working at desk jobs, who don't have much time for exercise. Simply exercise right at your desk (when the boss isn't looking).

Good luck!

Energy Tool

#47. Jin Shin Do (Acupressure Point Pressing)

In the 6,000-year-old Chinese Medicine system, there are over 350 acupuncture/acupressure points to press for more energy, situated on 14 "meridians" (networks of flowing chi-energy). Because it's extremely time-consuming to locate and press all 350 of these energizing points, an abbreviated system called Jin Shin Do was created, for quickly pressing about 38 ultra-key points, to energize your body in just 5 minutes!

An internet search of "Jin Shin Do points chart" only gives some "jin shin jyutsu" points (which work well, too) to look at, so in order to get and work with the 38 key points of authentic Jin Shin Do, you'll need to buy one of three books on Jin Shin Do by Iona Marsaa Teeguarden (available on the internet).

Once you learn (somewhat accurately) where the 38 points are, press them frequently for bodily energization! Experiment with this. Especially, in the morning when you get up, a 5-minute energizing-pressing-of-points really helps to get you going. It's also very effectively done during breaks at work, to quickly re-energize you! (Although, at work, you might need to retire to the privacy of a restroom stall, or your car in the parking lot, to do the pressing of these 38 key points for instant bodily energizing.)

Try it. This really works!

Energy Tool

#48. Laughing For Energy

Laughing makes you feel so genuinely good! And, you feel re-energized again. It's a great "internal exercise" for your lungs, diaphragm, and other organs too. Laughter makes you feel happy in a healthy, natural way. It's truly a great remedy for any "low energy blues" you might occasionally have.

Here is what you can try: every morning when you wake up, laugh for one minute. Move, gyrate, or roll your body around in bed (or do this standing up) in any way that works for you, to facilitate this (belly?) laughter. Try "laughing your brains out". Think of your favorite jokes (even if off-color). At first, your laughter may seem forced, but eventually, with practice, your daily laughter will grow stronger, and it will sound, and be, more genuine!

After practicing your 1-minute morning laughter for 3 days, increase it up to 2 minutes. Then, after a week, do it for 3 minutes. Keep up this morning laughter, more and more, until you've eventually reached 5 minutes of truly enjoyable laughter, every morning!

Laughing regularly will change your life! Your energy, mood, attitude, and outlook on life will all change for the better, uplifting your spirits greatly throughout your whole day. Laughter is such a great "energy remedy", facilitating your feeling "super" all over. Don't forget that you can laugh in the middle of the day too, or any time that you feel you really need it.

So, try it! Begin your every day with energizing, joyous, happy-making laughter!

Energy Tool

#49. Longan Fruit: Heart And Digestive Tonic

In Chinese Medicine (6,000 years old) there are a few dozen herbs that tonify various parts of the body. These tonic herbs are like vitamins that nourish and fortify the body. An example is ginseng, one of the most commonly known of these tonifying herbs.

Longan fruit is especially useful in tonifying the heart and digestive system. Longan can be bought fresh, as actual fruit, in some outdoor markets. Or you can visit a Chinese Herbalist and buy a big bag of dried (and preserved) longan fruit, to gradually eat over time.

Longan also has the advantage of being sweet and tasty to eat.

Since strengthening the heart and digestive system is so important, be sure to try longan. Then put it on your list of very effective energy tools, to eat (and tonify yourself) regularly!

Energy Tool

#50. Lymph Massage

We have a second system of fluid-filled tubes (besides the arteries and veins, filled with blood, and pumped by the heart). This second system is called the Lymph System, full of lymph fluid, and connected (in its network) to a multitude of lymph nodes. This lymph fluid flows to all our cells, to carry away waste. It's also an important part of our immune system.

What moves the lymph system, gradually throughout our body, is bodily motion. That's why a certain amount of exercise is important, to healthily move this lymph, in vessels, all around our body.

Also very important, in enabling lymph fluid to circulate, is massage of the lymph nodes and lymph vessels. This is called Lymph Massage.

You don't need to be a professional to do an effective lymph massage on yourself! Simply get a chart, or diagram, of the Lymph System (from the internet), and massage along the lymph channels, the best you can, in the direction of the large intestine (which the Lymph System empties into). Articles on the internet, along with a Lymph System diagram, will help get you started, here.

Especially when coming down with a cold, it helps greatly to massage the lymph system, for faster healing.

Regularly jumping up and down on a mini-rebounder (small trampoline) greatly helps to get the Lymph System flowing better, too! (See Energy Tool #55.)

All this will give you more energy, by making all your cells healthier, by facilitating the elimination of your cell waste products by your Lymph System. Try it!

Energy Tool

#51. Massage of Joints

Obviously, as people age, their joints stiffen up and become less fluid, more and more. The solution to this is to regularly massage all the joints in your body! This can result in a middle-aged person feeling and moving more like a teenager. Also, this can result in an older person feeling and moving more like a middle-aged person! See, the goal of joint massage is to limber up stiff joints so that people can "move more like a cat". So, how about it? Are you ready to start "moving more like a cat"?

"Fingertip Shiatsu" is the massage technique that accomplishes this. This type of massage involves making little circular finger movements as you press your fingertips into all the little indentations and "fleshy crevasses" where your joints are. Experiment with pressure, movement, and technique with your fingers, as you feel the resulting sensations in your joints!

Try doing this on the 15 finger joints on each hand. Then try the wrists, elbows, and shoulders of each arm. Doesn't it feel really good? Now do the ankles, knees, and hip joints. (It's hardest of all to penetrate your fingertips into these hip joints.)

The best way to massage the hip joints is to put the heel of your left hand over your left hip joint, then reach your right hand over to put your right hand over your left hand. Then, pull with your right hand, which results in pressure of the heel of your left hand going into your left hip joint. As you do this, make little circular movements with the heel of your left hand. Then do a mirror image of all this, to do your right hip.

Next, gently and carefully do the joints in your neck. Be very careful here!

Lastly, very carefully and gently do the vertebrae joints in your back. Here you might try my "Back Roller Massager (Energy Tool #9) or a Theracane (available on the internet).

After all your joints are massaged (perhaps eventually very rapidly in just 10 or 15 minutes), go ahead and walk around and feel how wonderful it feels to be so limber and loosened up in all your joints! You'll find that you feel younger and more energetic too, because all the blocks to your "flowing chi-energy" have been greatly reduced.

After trying all this, you'll probably never want to go back to being all "stiff-jointed" again! Especially, when all it takes is a quick 5-, or 10-, or 15-minute joint massage to make your joints and body feel great, so much younger, and more energized!

Energy Tool

#52. Meditation: Soothing, Restful, With Mantra

Profound rest of the body results in energy (afterward, when the rest is over). It's the Law of Yin and Yang. Extreme rest (Yin) eventually results in energy and action (Yang). Normally, a good night's sleep provides enough rest for getting active again the next day. But nowadays many Americans aren't getting enough sleep. They're just too busy! This is where meditation comes in, to greatly help to compensate for any shortage of sleep!

The brain waves in meditation (theta brain waves) are almost exactly like the brain waves of restful sleep (delta brain waves). Thus, meditation is very much like a nap; or perhaps more like a "waking nap", since you're still (barely) awake while meditating.

Instructions For Restful Meditation:

Sit in a comfortable chair, relax, close your eyes, and say out loud the mantra-sound "I-Ying", in as soothing a way as possible. Keep saying it over and over for perhaps 30 seconds. Then start saying it internally, inside your head (instead of out loud). Keep saying (in your head) "I-Ying", over and over, for 20 minutes. After these 20 minutes, the profound rest from the very soothed (theta) brain wave rhythms should make you feel refreshed, rested, and energized again (much like a successful nap).

Wearing ear plugs (optional) helps you to not be bothered by outer distracting noises. Also, you can meditate with I-Ying for lesser time periods. Even saying (internally) I-Ying for just 1 minute, or 2 minutes, or 5 minutes gives you a little rest and relief from stress (and eventually a little more energy).

Incidentally, the mantra I-Ying came to me intuitively while contemplating the yin-yang symbol. I realized that there is a relaxed, aware, "state of balance" between the "yang" state of Being (more active) and the "yin" state of Being (more passive). In trying to name this intermediate state, I realized that, in switching from the word "yang" and going to the word "yin", one first changes the "a" into an "i" and gets "ying". Then one drops the "g" and gets "yin". Similarly, in going back from "yin" to "yang", one adds a "g" and gets "ying". Then, one changes the "i" to an "a", and gets "yang".

Thus, "ying" is the intermediate, balanced state between yin and yang! But then, when meditating, instead of saying (the rather cumbersome) "I am ying", one abbreviates it into the simple "I Ying", or I-Ying. After my realization, when I experimented with internally repeating this mantra I-Ying, it worked superbly well in putting me into the deep, restful, balanced, profoundly meditative state that I was seeking. So, please consider trying this for yourself.

Saying I-Ying while lying in bed works well too, but can often result in you falling asleep! (Thus, it's a wonderful insomnia cure.) So, set your alarm clock for 20 minutes forward, if you can't risk falling asleep due to a future appointment.

Other mantras (besides I-Ying) can be used instead, but these other mantras must be soothing and relaxing to you, in order to have a similar restful effect. Repeating softly to yourself the word "relax" (with eyes closed) can be quite effective, too!

Saying I-Ying internally can even be done while walking in the world, with your eyes open. The effects of this are much more subtle, due to your open eyes and movement, but it still makes you feel more relaxed and less stressed. Wearing green color therapy glasses works well here for "open-eyed I-Ying saying" while walking. Obviously, don't say I-Ying while driving, because you always need to be very alert, to avoid accidents.

At work, it might be possible to get in 5 minutes (or so) of meditation, by retiring to the restroom and sitting (hidden away) in one of the stalls. (Could this be jokingly called "Ninja Meditation"?)

If you find that it's very hard for you to stay focused on the mantra, and daydreams constantly tend to "take over", then try tape recording I-Ying (said over and over for 20 minutes in your own voice). Then, when meditating, play back your 20-minute tape, which should help to reduce the daydreams and relax you more into profound, deep rest. (You could also tape-record your soothingly saying "relax" for 20 minutes, instead.) The result of this very relaxed rest will cause you to have more energy, when you finally come out of meditation!

Remember: profound relaxed rest (Yin) results, eventually, in more energy (Yang)!

Energy Tool

#53. Mega-Mag 400 Milligram.

This liquid magnesium (and 72 trace minerals) supplement works amazingly well to give you energy, perhaps because it really effectively penetrates all your cells.

Since most of us are magnesium (and trace mineral) deficient, this supplement is very important. It greatly relaxes and energizes you, while giving you that "feeling-good" experience, instantly!

It's available online at www.traceminerals.com, or by phoning them at (801) 731-6051 (or probably at your nearest health food store).

Try it!

Energy Tool

#54. Meridian Stroking For Energy

6,000 years ago, the ancient Chinese discovered a network of "energy tube channels" in the human body and called them "meridians". This was re-discovered in the West in 1937 and written up in an official medical journal, but doctors mostly ignored it. Sir Thomas Lewis of England published his report of discovery in the British Medical Journal of February 1937. He reported that his newly discovered system was composed of a network of incredibly minute lines. (See Chang's "The Book of Internal Exercises", pp. 8-9, which is Energy Tool #12.)

There are 12 main energy channels in the body, and they bring energy (or in Chinese, "chi") to all parts of the body. By hand-stroking (fairly hard) these 12 main energy-channel-meridians, you circulate energy around your body to all your vital organs, and feel energized again, and great!

The ancient Chinese found that all physical diseases and emotional stresses (!) are caused by blockages in the meridian energy flow (usually due to chronic muscular tension/Reichian body armor, which in turn is usually caused by traumatic emotional scarring from one's past). By getting the meridian energy flowing again (despite this bodily tension due to past emotional traumas) you'll feel vitality and happiness again. In fact, you might even start feeling yourself to be a bit younger, too!

Thus, by re-energizing yourself with re-flowing meridian energy, you'll feel revitalized and happier again, despite any lingering subconscious tension or emotional duress. (It's similar to the "feel-good" feeling after a good massage.)

Directions:

1. With your left palm facing up, place the "heel" of your right palm on your left shoulder (front deltoid muscle, at the top of it). Now, pressing down fairly hard, stroke this right hand's "heel" down your left arm, over the bicep, forearm, wrist, upright left palm, and upturned fingers. This fairly hard stroke should take about 2 seconds. Then, lift up your right hand's "heel", and lifting it off of your left hand's fingers, return it through the air (not touching the left arm) to where you began. Do this complete stroke, down the upturned left arm, 3 more times.

2. Then do the mirror-image, i.e., the same thing with the other arm, using the left hand's "heel" to stroke (4 times) down the upturned right arm, in the same way, from the top of the

shoulder to the upturned fingers. You've now energetically stroked 3 of the main 12 meridians: the lung meridian, the heart meridian, and the pericardium (heart-protecting) meridian. If you want, you can look up these 3 meridians on the internet, and see that their path of "acupuncture chi points" does indeed go down the inside of your 2 arms, which you've just energetically stroked!

3. Now, turn your left palm over, facing down (so that you can see your fingernails). Place the "heel" of your right hand over the left hand's knuckles, and stroke up (fairly hard) with your right hand's "heel". First over the back of the wrist, up to the elbow, then (from the elbow) going to the back (or tricep) part of the left arm. Stroke up along your tricep to your left arm's rear deltoid muscle. This stroke should be continuous (not pausing too much at the elbow) and should take about 2 seconds. Then, lift the heel of your right hand through the air (not touching the left arm) and back to your left hand's knuckles again. Do this stroke (fairly hard) 3 more times, in the same way. It works even better, here, if, when your stroke gets past your elbow, to switch to pressing your tricep hard with your fisted knuckles (instead of your hand's "heel"). Your fisted knuckles will then be able to exert much more pressure, as they slide up along your tricep.

4. Then do the mirror-image same thing with the other arm, using your left hand's "heel" to stroke 4 times up the "palm-facing-down" right arm. You've now energetically stroked 3 more of the main 12 meridians: the small intestine meridian, the large intestine meridian, and the "triple warmer" meridian (which influences your endocrine system). If you want, you can look up these 3 meridians on the internet, and see that their path of "acupuncture chi points" does indeed go up the outside of your arms.

   Do you feel slightly more energized in your upper body now? Doesn't it feel good?

5. Now place the "heel" of your right palm on the inside of your left ankle bone. Stroke the "heel" of your right palm up the inside of your left leg, to your upper thigh, taking about 3 seconds with this stroke. Then move your right hand's "heel" through the air (not touching your leg) back to your left ankle, and stroke up, like before, 3 more times.

6. Then do the mirror-image same thing with the other leg, stroking up with the "heel" of your left hand, from the inside of your right leg's ankle, up the inside of your leg, to the inside of your upper thigh. Do this stroke 4 times too. You've just

energized the kidney meridian, the liver meridian, and the spleen meridian. (Look up these 3 meridians on the internet, if you want.)

7. Now place both "heels" of your palms on your hip bones, on the outside of your 2 legs. Pressing fairly hard, stroke your hand's "heels" down the outside of your 2 legs, to the outer ankle bones of your feet. Do this 4 times. This energizes the gallbladder meridian. (Look it up on the internet, if you want.)

8. Now place both "heels" of your palms on the top middle of your thighs, and (pressing fairly hard), stroke down the top of your thighs, over your knees, and down your shins, to the beginning of your feet. Do this 4 times. This energizes the stomach meridian. (Look it up.)

9. Now, place the knuckles of your hands under your upper thighs (where the thighs meet your buttocks). Slide the knuckles of your hands down the underside of your thighs, behind your knees, across the back of your calves, and down to the heels of your feet. Do this 4 times. This energizes the bladder meridian. (Look it up on the internet, if you want.)

10. Now repeat point 3. again.

11. Now repeat point 1. again.

12. Now repeat point 2. again.

You're done! You've just energized all 12 meridians, so that your meridian chi-energy is flowing a lot more strongly, making you feel more vitalized and happy. Feel it? You can do this technique as much as you want, to energize yourself and feel good, because it's a natural, healthy way to feel high! Also, now that you've learned it, it should go much faster in the future, to where it should only take about 3 to 5 minutes to do!

P.S. Doing this technique too close to your bedtime may result in insomnia. You might give yourself so much energy that you can't get to sleep! So, watch this. Perhaps don't do it within 3 or 4 hours of your bedtime? Experiment with this, so that you find the "cutoff" time, here.

Energy Tool

#55. Mini-Rebounder

This very helpful device is a circular, 6-foot diameter, mini-trampoline, on which you (gently ?) jump up and down. In fact, there's a whole exercise regimen you can do on it, if you want.

But, the most important thing it does is to stimulate your lymph fluid, and to get it flowing more efficiently through your body. See, your lymph fluid system is similar to the blood flow in your circulatory system, but it has no pump (no "heart") to pump the lymph fluid. The main reason your blood circulates and nourishes all your cells with oxygen and nutrients (and takes away waste) is because of your heart's pumping action. But there's no "pump" in the lymph fluid system.

Instead, valuable lymph fluid circulation is caused by your bodily motion! This is where the mini-rebounder really helps. Jumping up and down (and all around) on your mini-rebounder does wonders in circulating valuable lymph fluid to all your cells.

Of course, active aerobic exercise also helps to circulate lymph fluid, but jumping on a mini-rebounder does it even better!

Once more of your lymph fluid is circulating, all your cells will be significantly healthier, to then produce more energy, for a more energetic you!

Energy Tool

#56. Minimize (Or Stop) Caffeine

Caffeine is a stimulant drug, as opposed to a tonic. It's extremely important to understand the huge difference between tonics and stimulant-drugs, here!

Tonics are vitamins and herbs that nourish the body in a healthy, supportive way. For example, ginseng and about 25 other tonic herbs from the Chinese Medicine System are very nurturing and supportive to the body. Most of these tonic herbs are described in Ron Teegarten's book "Chinese Tonic Herbs", available on the internet. All the vitamins are healthy tonics, too. Reishi mushroom capsules, Cordyceps mushroom capsules, and Shiitake mushroom capsules (all tonics) are also tremendously nourishing to the body, and give lots of energy. Basically, all tonics are very good for the body, and give you an "energy high" without any following "energy low".

Stimulant-drugs, on the other hand, are usually bad for the body! In the typical drug-way, these stimulants "seem" to give you energy in the short run, but always give fatigue and exhaustion in the long run! Stimulant-drugs (and even tea and guarana, which have the drug caffeine) push the body harshly, forcing it unhealthily into action, catalytically tapping your reserve energies, in the short run. But, when these reserve energies are diminished and depleted, exhaustion and fatigue result, in the long run. Always, with any drug this happens: the "drug high" later results in a "drug low" (which then feels pretty rotten).

Why put yourself through the "drug high", then awful "drug low" process with stimulant-drugs, when instead you can have the "tonic high" without any "tonic low"? That's right, tonics (unlike stimulant-drugs) give an "energy high" without any "energy low" later on! So, why keep taking stimulant-drugs with their horrible eventual "drug low", when you can switch to tonics and thus totally avoid any eventual "low"? Doesn't this make far more sense?

So, the choice here is rather crystal-clear, isn't it? Take tonics instead of stimulant-drugs! (Which includes the caffeine stimulant-drugs of coffee and tea.)

Energy Tool

#57. Minimize (Or Stop) Drugs

Most drugs are really poisons that your body tries to eliminate through your liver and kidneys (straining them considerably). Also, antibiotic drugs can kill off the helpful probiotic bacteria in your small intestine, that help digest and assimilate food. All this reduces your energy levels.

Thus, keep drugs to an absolute minimum. Try using more healing herbs, instead of drugs. Begin trying to be your own healer, with herbs and alternative therapies. Learn from any friends you have who are already doing this. Have your friends teach you any alternative remedies that they know of (or, find and take classes in this).

Using more natural-remedy healing techniques and less drug-poison medicine seems the way to go, to maximize your health and bodily energy. So, try to slowly transition, here, if you can!

Energy Tool

#58. Moonlight (Reversed With Mirror) Soul Healing

Many stories abound, regarding moonlight making people feel "crazier". The full moon (Luna) can especially make you feel like an utter lunatic! This is because the moon acts as a mirror to reflect light from the sun toward the earth. Thus, moonlight is "reversed sunlight", or the opposite of the sun's healthy, warm, revitalizing energy. This reflected opposite, or "negative sunlight" energy from the moon is what disorients and confuses people who gaze too much at the moon at night.

But, what if you held up a good-sized mirror at night, angled so that you were gazing at the moon reflected in your mirror (instead of moon-gazing directly)? Then, the mirror would serve to reverse the moonlight back into sunlight, right? Light from the sun would reverse on the moon, then reverse again in your mirror, before it hits your eyes, as "original" sunlight again, right?

When I experimented many times, with gazing at the moon (at night) through a mirror, I've found repeatedly that reversed moonlight acts like a kind of "mild sunlight", in healing my soul!

Yes! Somehow, the doubly reflected light from the sun (first reflected off the moon, then reflected again off your mirror to your eyes) energizes, soothes, heals, and revitalizes you, deeply, at a soul level! I greatly encourage you to experience this for yourself, firsthand!

The wonderful thing about gazing at the moon at night through a mirror is that it's a similar energy to the sun. But since it's been doubly reflected, it's much easier on your eyes, to look at for quite some time. Anyway, try it! But if the reflected moonlight starts to feel too intense, either to your eyes or to your soul, then draw your "mirror-reversed moon gazing" to a close, until perhaps the next night. You might need to go slow with this Energy Tool!

P.S. Instead of a mirror, you can soulfully and energizingly gaze at reflected moonlight in a river, a lake, a swimming pool, the ocean, a puddle left by rainwater, the water in a filled-up 5-gallon bucket, a hand-held bowl or pot of water, or even the moist dew on forest plants glistening exotically in the nighttime moonlight (especially after a recent rainfall). Experiment with all this, and deeply, soulfully enjoy it!

Energy Tool

#59. Mushrooms Of Power

There are 3 great mushroom supplements to take:

- Reishi Mushroom,
- Cordyceps Mushroom,
- Shitake Mushroom.

In a very thorough and definitive book on mushrooms entitled "Mycelium Running: How Mushrooms Can Help Save The World", by Paul Stamets, dozens of mushrooms are mentioned, but the above 3 appear to be the very best, in giving you the most energy and other healthful benefits.

Do a search on these 3 mushrooms on the internet, and familiarize yourself with all their multiple health benefits. Consider taking them regularly (in capsule form) to then have more energy in your life!

Energy Tool

#60. Nam Myoho Renge Kyo

In Japan, there is a big organization of people who chant "Nam Myoho Renge Kyo". "Nam" in Japanese means "devotion". "Myoho" means "mystic law". "Renge" means "cause and effect". And "Kyo" means "enlightened teaching of Buddha".

Thus, this entire chant means something like "I devote myself to the mystic law of cause and effect, according to the enlightened teaching of my Higher (Buddha-like) Self".

A little thinking about the "Law of Cause and Effect" discloses that it's a very important law to follow (devotedly?) indeed! Another way to say it is "As ye sow, so shall ye reap". In other words, "a wise plan and action often leads to a successful and happy result", whereas a stupid plan (or no plan) with laziness (or little action or wrong action) often leads to failure and unhappiness. Furthermore, "good cause often leads to good effect", and "bad cause often leads to bad effect". (The word "often" is in here because the "luck factor" can play a part in this, too. Also, you can sometimes be swindled by unfairness, accidents, con men, thieves, or by lying, deceitful other people, etc.)

Tony Robbins and others like him (in their empowerment seminars and books) advocate "taking charge" of your life. This basically means deliberately putting yourself at "good cause", in order to produce and experience a "good effect" in your life, as much as possible!

Chanting "Nam Myoho Renge Kyo" energizes you psychologically and emotionally, I've found, to motivate you to stop procrastinating and "get out there and do it". Thus, those things that you know you need to do (to create a more successful and happier life) actually get done, with the help of this chant. Other chants exist, of course; that may work too. Or, you could even try creating your own chant, here. But, I've personally found that the chant "Nam Myoho Renge Kyo" works for me (to get the job done) better than any other chant!

Try this chant. It really seems to work well, to "get you going". It strongly motivates you to take action!

In addition, surprisingly, there often occurs a secondary effect from a lot of chanting, namely: more luck! Somehow, favorable "coincidences" seem to occur more often, due to your chanting; these help out your life progress even more than your "smart work" does by itself!

Energy Tool

#61. Naps

If you're able to actually fall asleep for a while, in the middle of the day, then do it! For, this short nap really rests your body well. It's like a little "siesta", and will result in more energy, plus less sleep required during the night.

Most of us have heard the story of Thomas Edison and his taking several short naps during the day so that he only had to sleep 3 to 4 hours at night. Thus, Eddison "swore by" his naps.

Yes, naps do work to rest and energize, but some have trouble with the "groggy feeling" which can often persist after waking up from an afternoon nap. In fact, sometimes this "groggy feeling" is so annoying and persistent that it completely wrecks the effectiveness of naps altogether! (You might try rocking passionately in a rocking chair, right after your nap, to offset this. See Energy Tool #73. Or, after the nap, you could press the 3 acupressure "points of power", to give you a great burst of energy. See Energy Tool #1. Or, you could take 5 capsules of cordyceps mushrooms. See Energy Tool #59.)

Anyway, consider experimenting with naps at different times in the day, and of different duration, to try to find a type of nap that works for you, and is then well worth doing regularly, to give your body more energy.

Energy Tool

#62. Nature Walk

Nature is our true home. For hundreds of thousands of years, our species lived totally in nature, and developed our whole physiology based on this nature living. It's so easy to forget this when we're so used to living in a concrete, steel, plastic, and glass "artificial" world.

In nature, we relax, exercise, and get fresh air. Our endorphins are enhanced by returning to the natural world, where our whole species evolved and began. Just feeling and experiencing how good we feel in nature is reason enough to take regular nature walks. It's a great way to re-energize us, too!

Nature walks also give us a fresh perspective on our life and its issues. New solutions can intuitively appear, as we walk.

Be sure to make time for an occasional excursion into nature. You'll be very glad you did!

Perhaps, singing Don Ho's song "Take a Walk in the Country" periodically will help you to remember the importance of nature walks.

Energy Tool

#63. Ocean Healing (Water Therapy)

If you're living by the ocean, or by a lake, river, pond, or stream, getting in the water can really make you feel "cleaned out", refreshed, and rejuvenated. Your energy afterward can feel markedly more healthy!

Hot tubs, swimming pools, baths, and even showers can do this, too, to some extent.

Take advantage of "water therapy" and the "power of water", to clean out your "aura" and "negative energy", so that you'll have a refreshed and rejuvenated experience, with more and better energy, afterward.

Doing this regularly really helps you to feel healthier, and more energetic!

P.S. Obviously, all toxins and poisons (in the environment and in your diet) need to be avoided and distanced from, since they can all drastically reduce your energy! However, any toxins or poisons that still remain can be cleaned out of you, by ocean healing and water therapy (which is why this type of therapy is so important!)

Energy Tool

#64. Ocean Surf Walk And Negative Ion Therapy

When ocean waves reach the shore and break on the sand, enormous numbers of negative ions are released into the air. Well, breathing these negative ions makes you feel "high", and re-energizes you!

If you're lucky enough to live relatively close to the ocean, you can schedule regular ocean visits into your busy life. Then you can enjoy a "barefoot wading" through the ocean surf, as you exhilaratingly inhale all these healthy negative ions!

Waterfalls, too, give off lots of negative ions, when the water (falling down from up high) crashes into the pool of water below. If you can safely get near the base of the waterfall, you can (very enjoyably) breathe in negative ions at that spot. Also, to a certain extent, your shower can be regarded as a "mini-waterfall". As the shower water crashes down onto the concrete floor of your shower stall, negative ions are released there. By sitting on the floor of your shower stall (or sitting on a very short-legged wood stool in the shower stall) you can breathe in the negative ions accumulating at the bottom of your shower stall. After taking your regular shower, experimentally try this! (You might need to keep the floor of your shower stall extremely clean, using a non-toxic organic cleaning solution, with no toxic chemical odors. This way no mold, germs, dirty fumes, or bad chemical vapors will be breathed in along with the healthy negative ions.)

Negative Ion Generators exist too, for this purpose, and you might also be interested in investigating this further.

Anyway, arrange to breathe in these negative ions (if possible) and experience the re-energizing effects for yourself. Then you'll be more motivated to regularly do this, once you've found out how good it makes you feel!

Energy Tool

#65. Palming Eyes With Hands

In the Bates System of eye re-education, which has several exercises to gradually improve your eyesight, there is one technique that's called "palming".

In "palming", you place your left open palm over your left eye, and your right open palm over your right eye. The palms are there simply to shut out light, and give a sensation of darkness to your eyes, so that your eyes can (profoundly) rest.

It works! After palming, your eyes do feel more rested. Palming can be done for just 30 seconds, 1 minute, 5 minutes, 20 minutes, or even longer. Usually, the longer you do the palming, the more profoundly rested your eyes feel afterward.

Also, when you finish your palming, you feel rested and refreshed in your body and emotions too, and thus you'll feel more energized, as a result.

Try it! Refresh and re-energize yourself with palming, especially if you're either stressed or exhausted. You can combine this palming with Energy Tool #52 (Meditation: Soothing, Restful, With Mantra), for even better results, here. Go for it!

Energy Tool

#66. Peripheral Vision

Most people pay almost exclusive attention to the visual field that's right in front of their eyes. This "front-vision-field" tends to be what they mostly focus on, throughout their day.

But instead, you can consciously and deliberately put your attention on your peripheral vision (while your eyes are still looking forward into the distance). In other words, physically your eyes are looking forward still, but mentally you're focusing on objects perceived in your peripheral vision (to your left, to your right, up above, and down below). The effect of this is to wake you up (out of your ego), to give you more perspective! Insights can occur here, that can be really helpful, in improving the quality of your life. You'll find this out, when you try it!

See, we become so ultra-focused, with our "tunnel-visioned" ego, that we tend to lose perspective of what's truly important, and what's not (and often only blind habit).

So, peripheral vision (employed briefly, once in a while) gives us energy to re-evaluate what's really top-priority in our lives and what's not!

Feel free to employ this peripheral-vision-awakening tool several times, briefly, during your day. But you might need to keep it brief (only 3 seconds?) at first, in case it tends to strain your eyes' peripheral vision fields too much, initially. So experiment, keep the "peripheralizing" brief at first, and see how well it works for you!

Energy Tool

#67. Pow Wow Step

When I tried the "American Indian Pow Wow Step" at gatherings of Native Americans, it really seemed to work! I felt lots more energy and enthusiasm, after Pow-Wow-Stepping around in a big circle, with a gathering of many others. The skillful, steady drumming, along with a high-pitched "wailing" song, really helped in this energizing process.

The way that you do the Pow Wow Step is rather simple. You move forward your left foot and touch just the toe to the ground. Quickly after that, you set the whole of your left foot onto the ground. Then you do the exact same thing with your right foot. And that's it! These are the steps:

(1) Toe-touch (only) with left foot,

(2) Step entire left foot onto the ground,

(3) Toe-touch (only) with right foot, and

(4) Step entire right foot onto the ground.

Etc. Over and over, while walking in a big circle! (Do a search on the internet if you need more instruction or explanation, here.)

Probably, over many thousands of years, many tribes of Native Americans developed this powerful Pow Wow Tool, as a means of energizing, re-inspiring, and reducing depression by a process of "wailing out their sorrows of a life filled with an almost endless struggle for survival". The intense, skillful drumming and group energy helps greatly in this process, too.

In the past, Native Americans, along with many other ancient peoples, led a very hard and harsh life. If too much depression and angst accumulated from this struggle-to-survive, it was extremely helpful to release it, in a large wailing/drumming/pow-wow-stepping gathering! Similarly, in your own life (filled with a certain amount of stress) it can be extremely helpful to release this stress by doing the Pow-Wow-Step on a regular basis. Right? Also, it's all rather fun, once you get the hang of it!

Anyway, try it! It can be done inside your place, or outside in your yard, or at a park somewhere, etc. Pow Wow CD music (of drumming and "wailing") can be purchased on the internet, which greatly helps facilitate this whole energizing-and-releasing process, for you.

It'll feel so good, during and after, that you'll probably want to experience "doing the Pow-Wow-Step" more than once!

Energy Tool

#68. Power Crystal Hold

Crystals have power and energy! But since there are hundreds (or even thousands) of crystals to hold and get energy from, you'll have to experiment with many, to find the right empowering crystal for you!

Perhaps start with quartz crystals, which many books say contain great power and energy. Surf through the internet, searching for energizing and empowering (or healing) crystals. Buy informative books on crystals. Better yet, visit a crystal shop, or crystal booth at a swap meet. Vibe out many of the crystals there, by holding them, to experience what feels good to you.

It's well worth your time, to find just the right empowering and energizing (or healing) crystal that works especially well for you.

So, make it happen!

Energy Tool

#69. Probiotics And Prebiotics

What goes on in your gut (small intestine) is a lot more important than people used to think! Firstly, quality digestion, of transforming food into energy, should be happening there. And secondly, multitudes of friendly/helpful bacteria should be helping this super-digestive process, while reducing and eliminating the bad bacteria (which foul things up).

Probiotics is essentially fortifying your gut by ingesting billions of the "good guy"-friendly/helpful bacteria, who will then help digestion and kill off the "bad guy" bacteria. And, prebiotics is eating the foods that nourish the "good guy" bacteria, once they're "doing their job", in your gut!

When digestion greatly improves, with probiotics and prebiotics, you'll then have much more energy to use to create a happier and more successful life. You'll feel a lot healthier in your gut, too, which also contributes to a more energized, happy, and successful you!

So, consider experimenting with the various probiotic and prebiotic products at your local health food store. Also, learning more about all this from the internet, books, and DVDs, helps greatly.

Energy Tool

#70. Pulling And Swishing Fluid In Your Mouth

Oil swishing and "pulling" is where you put a small amount of oil in your mouth and do swishing and "pulling" mouth movements. It thoroughly cleans your mouth of germs, and also tends to "pull" out toxins from your gum tissue. It's excellent for teeth and gum health, and also gives you more energy by expelling toxins (first from your gums, then gradually from your whole body).

An internet search on "oil pulling" will fill you in on its numerous benefits, etc. Books on "oil pulling" can be bought and learned from, too. It's extremely popular in India.

I started out using vegetable oil, then later coconut oil, and still later filtered tap water! Filtered water works about 80% as well as oil, and filtered water is so cheap that it's practically free. Also, swishing water doesn't require brushing your teeth afterward, to rid your mouth of the "oily taste". Plus, swished and pulled water is easy to dispose of. Just spit it out into the sink! Whereas spitting *oil* into your sink is very unwise, because it will eventually clog up your plumbing. Instead, spit the oil into a disposable container (like an empty milk carton, etc.) and then dispose of this container in the trash. Don't ever swallow the water or oil that you've just swished, or you'll just be swallowing all your own swished out germs and toxins. (But if you do accidentally swallow a little, it won't really be all that bad for you. Just try to avoid swallowing most of it.)

Swishing or "pulling" water (or oil) in your mouth exercises your mouth muscles quite a bit, so that at first your swishing sessions may be brief. But gradually, your mouth muscles will strengthen.

My own technique for "pulling" water in my mouth is to do it "sectionally" in 6 different mouth locations, one section after another. This is much easier on the mouth muscles, and greatly reduces "mouth muscle strain".

(1) First, swish and "pull" the water in the upper left section of your mouth (only), over your left upper teeth and gums.

(2) Next, swish and "pull" the water in the upper middle part of your mouth (only), over your middle upper teeth and gums.

(3) Then swish and "pull" the water in the upper right section of your mouth (only), over your upper right teeth and gums.

(4) Now swish and "pull" the water in the lower right section of your mouth (only), over your lower right teeth and gums.

(5) Then swish and "pull" the water in the lower middle part of your mouth (only), over your lower middle teeth and gums.

(6) Lastly, swish and "pull" the water in the lower left section of your mouth (only), over your lower left teeth and gums.

(7) Now spit out the germy-tasting water, take another large sip of new water, and do it all again! (Unless your mouth muscles are just so exhausted that you need to stop, here.)

Eventually, your mouth muscles will strengthen enough to do this whole 6-part sequence for 3 entire times! Then you'll be rewarded by feeling your mouth to be cleaner than you've ever experienced before!

Anyway, it works well to give you more energy, after all these germs and toxins are swished and "pulled" out of your mouth, and disappear down the drain. Try it!

Energy Tool

#71. Reflexology (Feet)

Massaging all the reflexology points on the soles of your feet gives you lots(!) of energy in the corresponding organs and parts of your body. Using a wooden foot-roller-massager, place your foot on it (on the floor), and roll your foot back and forth over it, to your heart's content! (But caution here: be sure to pick up the wooden roller off the floor afterward, or someone could trip over it and have an accidental fall!)

You can create your very own foot-roller-massager by buying a 1 1/4 inch diameter dowel at the hardware store, then sawing off two 6 inch lengths from it (one for each foot). With practice, you can effectively massage both feet at the same time, using both wooden foot rollers at once!

Look on the internet for more advanced, grooved wooden foot-roller-massagers.

Rolling your feet regularly on your 2 wooden foot-roller-massagers works to energize you, by stimulating all the reflexology points in your feet that correspond to all the organs in your body. In other words, as you massage your feet, you energize your body's organs at the same time!

There are several books on the internet that show you how to use foot massage and foot reflexology, to energize your whole body, in this way. Check them out!

By including foot massage, in your daily morning "wake up" regimen, it may really work to energize you in the morning. Try it!

P.S. Once again, be absolutely certain that you don't negligently leave a wooden foot-roller-massager on the floor after use, or someone could trip over it and have an accidental fall! In fact, unless you're enough of a "perfectionist" to remember to always pick up the foot-roller-massager after use, it might be better (unfortunately) to not try using this Energy Tool. What you could try here, is (just before using the 2 foot-roller-massagers) to put a rubber band around each wrist! Then, when you're finished using the 2 foot-roller-massagers, the 2 rubber bands will be a very important reminder to pick up the 2 foot-roller-massagers off the floor and place them (and the 2 rubber bands) into a box on a nearby table, in a way so that the 2 foot-roller-massagers can't possibly get out of this box and fall onto the floor. Be sure to safeguard yourself with some kind of foolproof method like this! Also, if the phone rings, or someone rings your front doorbell while you're foot-roller-massaging, be absolutely certain to take the 2 foot-roller-massagers off the floor and put them into the box on the table, before answering the phone or the doorbell! Make this ultra-important to do!

Energy Tool

#72. Reflexology (Hands)

Reflexology is much more than pressing one little area on a hand reflexology chart, to improve the health of just one organ or part of your body. Instead, you can press all the reflexology points on the hand chart, over and over. And, do this as hard as you can stand it, too! By doing this, you'll be stimulating (abundantly) all the corresponding organs and areas in your body, to give you lots more energy. It really works!

One of the best books on this is "Health Is In Your Hands", by Devendra Vora. This very wise author has healed hundreds of people in India with his methods. His excellent book contains several more outstanding healing techniques, too!

So, if you want to utterly load yourself with energy, press (fairly hard) all the reflexology points on both hands, several times each day! Using a wooden "peg" or a "massage stick" helps a lot here, too. Either design your own wooden peg, dowel, or stick, or do a search on the internet for one to buy.

You can create your own simple massage stick (or peg) by buying a 1" diameter wooden dowel at the hardware store, Walmart, or Ben Franklin store. A 7/8" diameter dowel works well, too. Saw off the end to about 6" in length. Then use a high-quality file to round off one of the ends of this 6" peg, to be more like the rounded-off end of a broom's handle. (This is the most difficult part, and may take some time and patience to make it extremely smooth.) Then, grasping your 6" massage stick in one hand, massage your other palm with the rounded-off end of your massage stick. Using oil helps a lot, here (coconut oil is best). You'll find that massaging your hand's reflexology points is greatly facilitated by your own massage stick (or "peg"). It's possible to massage your palm's reflexology points with your other hand's knuckles and perhaps some saliva (for a lubricant) if you are needy for some "instant energy", but your best results (by far) will be achieved with your personal peg and some coconut oil lubricant.

Try it. You'll find that you'll be greatly energized by this!

Energy Tool

#73. Rocking Chair Power

Rocking chairs aren't just for old people. No! Instead, they're for people who really want to ROCK!

See, in a rocking chair you can rock so hard and so fast that your body almost feels like it's on a carnival ride. Really! And you know how much fun that can be!

Passionate rocking greatly helps in moving your lymph (and other bodily fluids, too), to promote health and energy. But I'm not getting into the physiology of this thing too much, here. All I know is that rocking feels great! And, the faster and harder you rock, the greater the benefits. Try it, and you'll see!

There's a book on the internet, "The Rocking Chair Exercise Book" by Dr. Henry F. Ogle. He has put together an entire (brief) daily exercise program, all done in a rocking chair. According to him, rocking even helps greatly in trimming the waistline!

Rocking is also a great way for run-down, fatigued people to get in a little healthy exercise, while markedly improving their lymph and bodily fluid systems.

Rocking chairs aren't even that expensive! And, rocking is such a great way to fully wake up in the morning (or from a nap). Or, even to have a stimulating conversation with your friends, as you both passionately rock away (each in your own rocking chair).

Anyway, it's well worth a try. Don't let any "cultural prejudice" stop you, from super-rocking yourself to more energy and health!

P.S. As you delightfully rock away, you can also watch T.V., or your computer, or DVDs. You can also make phone calls, listen to the radio, or even play your favorite rock music! Enjoy!

Energy Tool

#74. Roller-Massager-Tool Power!

So many of us have a lot of muscular tension! We could really use a bit of massage, to help relax ourselves more. The trouble is, most massage practitioners are expensive and also somewhat of a hassle to schedule a massage with. Right?

Self-massage can greatly help us here, but we need to learn "how". Also, self-massage tends to wear out our fingers too fast. In addition, there seems to be some kind of "social taboo" against doing self-massage; we're almost a little "embarrassed" about practicing it on ourselves, somehow.

This is why the Roller-Massage-Tool is so outstandingly useful! The Roller-Massager (easy-to-make-massage-tool) is simply a stick (14"-long dowel, 5/8"-diameter thickness) with 2 tennis balls, 2 "pinkie" balls, or 3 racquetballs on it.

Instructions For Making It:

- With an electric drill, drill a 5/8"-diameter hole in a tennis ball (puncturing in only about an inch, and not out the opposite side yet). Then, very carefully locating the spot exactly opposite your first hole, drill a second hole in the tennis ball. Great care must be used in very accurately locating the 180 degrees-opposite second hole, or the final 2-holed ball will "wobble" too much on the stick (when in use). Take a few minutes of time here, to very precisely locate this second hole!

- Drill the 2 holes in the second tennis ball in the same way as you did with the first ball. Then, shove the 2 (holed) tennis balls onto the stick, to reside in the exact middle of the stick. It helps also to screw on 2 little wood cylinders, outside the 2 tennis balls, to restrict the 2 balls to the exact middle of the stick (see picture). Two "pinkie" balls or 3 racquetballs can be used instead of the 2 tennis balls, here.

You now have your very own Roller-Massager-Tool, all ready for use. So, roll away! Try it on your arms, legs, lower back, under your feet, all over your scalp, on your buttocks, on your neck, on your shoulders, everywhere! Massaging your whole body with this tool not only feels wonderful, but it doesn't strain your fingers (like regular self-massage does).

Keep a Roller-Massager handy in your car, backpack, or purse, to use continually throughout your day. As your muscular tension is easily massaged away, you'll reduce your stress, feel great, and have more energy too.

Try it!

Energy Tool

#75. Sex

We all understand the importance of a great sex life, even if you are not in a relationship. Almost all of us have a sex drive to satisfy. But the main problem seems to be that many of us don't have (available) a compatible-enough partner who's willing to do it with us. And this is a very common lament, it seems!

Enter fantasy! Unfortunately, that's what we (very healthily) need to turn to, when reality (and a rather puritanical society) doesn't satisfy our healthy instinctual bodily needs!

Even though people are often very creative and resourceful when satisfying their financial, material, health-related, and recreational needs, when it comes to sexual needs, it's often done way too quickly and superficially. Because of embarrassment and social taboo (you can't talk about it), most people's self-sex is very far from fulfilling.

Mark Twain once quipped: "90% of people masturbate, and the other 10% are liars!" Doesn't this still hold true, even today?

"The Sensuous Woman", by "J" (the pen name of Terry Joan Garrity), and "The Sensuous Man", by "M" (the pen name of Joan, John Garrity, and Len Foreman), are great to read (along with many other books similar to these) for bringing more ecstasy, ultra-satisfaction, and even some "solo-tantra" into self-sex.

I'm sorry that this Energy-Tool needs to be included here (if any readers feel awkward about it), but how happy can a more-energized-you be, if your sexuality is frustrated and thwarted?

Energy Tool

#76. Shower With A Non-Pore-Clogging Soap

Unfortunately, most soaps have chemical additives that clog your pores too much. This is undesirable, because your skin pores actually take in a certain amount of oxygen, which increases your energy.

"Beyond" soap contains nothing that will clog your skin's pores and is available at Walmart, the last I heard.

"Filthy Farm Girl" soap also contains no additives, and is available at health food stores. (Or, on the internet.)

"Kiss My Face" soap used to contain nothing that would clog your skin's pores, but the old company was bought out by a new company that changed the formula. But at a health food store I was able to find a bar (still) of the old formula, which apparently continues to be available too.

By an internet search, you might find another soap that's "unclogging" to your skin's pores.

Maximize your energy by keeping your skin pores open, to take in oxygen. Switch to a soap that has no chemical additives in the soap (that clog your skin's pores). Then, try this new "unclogging" soap, and feel the difference!

Energy Tool

#77. Shungite, To Reduce "5G" EMF Radiation

EMF (Electro-Magnetic Field) radiation, which flows out from all electrical devices, reduces physical vitality. The more electrically powerful the device, the more EMF radiation flows out, and the more fatigue that's caused.

Especially with the upgrading of urban centers to "5G" (from "3G") is this a problem. Lectures that I attended provided much evidence that "5G" EMF radiation might be one hundred times as powerful, and damaging-to-your-health, as "3G" EMF radiation! Apparently, much greater health problems, of fatigue, headaches, muddled thinking, insomnia, and depression, etc., will result from massive city-wide "5G" EMF radiation. If you have lately been suffering from the above adverse symptoms (when you weren't so much before about 2017), perhaps it's the new "5G" EMF radiation (now in most big cities) that's the cause!

Shungite (a black mineral) greatly helps to reduce, cut down, and even stop EMF radiation. You can read about shungite's effectiveness on the internet, and perhaps even buy a book telling you all about shungite. You can order shungite bead-necklaces (to wear around outdoors, under your shirt), or 2" high black shungite pyramids to put between you and your computer or T.V., etc.

But you need an authentic source of shungite, for "con men" are selling black slate and black onyx on the internet, and falsely claiming that it's shungite! The authentic source for shungite is a woman in Oregon, whose phone number is (602) 292-6818. Or

karen@urielcreations.com, or www.urielcreations.com. Ask her about all the shungite devices she has in stock.

Good luck in using shungite as a tool to reduce fatigue, from "5G" and all other EMF radiation!

P.S. You can find many other methods and devices on the internet that protect you from EMF radiation.

Energy Tool

#78. Slapping (Lightly) All Over Your Body

There's a form of self-massage, very energizing, that involves gently slapping yourself all over your body. Try it first on your left arm and hand, slapping gently with your right open hand. Isn't it stimulating? Now, after slapping your left arm like this, pause a second and compare both arms. Doesn't your left arm feel more "alive", and your (unslapped as yet) right arm feel more "dead", or "asleep", by comparison?

Now slap your left arm again, harder (without it being too stinging) all over, then compare your two arms again. Get the point? Your left arm feels super-stimulated and energized, compared to the whole rest of your body. Right?

Proceed by (gently?) slapping your right arm and hand, then your legs and feet, then your chest and stomach, then your buttocks and back (as well as you can). Then slap your neck, face (more lightly) and head. Be slapped and energized all over, in this way.

Don't you now feel great, stimulated, and energized all over your whole body? Yes! This really works! And it usually takes only 5 minutes to do it all, if you're in a hurry and don't have much time. In fact, if you're in a super-hurry, you can rapidly slap yourself all over in just 1 minute! Isn't this incredible? Just 1 minute of slapping yourself all over your whole body, makes you feel this great and energized!

Apply this energizing slap-massage tool whenever you need some quick whole-body energy!

Energy Tool

#79. Sleeping Sufficiently

Sleep rejuvenates and refreshes your body, when you get the full 8 or 9 hours. It's the super-important nightly "yin" that balances the daily "yang". Sleep is almost a miracle in how it transforms your fatigue (from yesterday) to having energy again today!

Don't take sleep's miracle for granted. Appreciate it, instead. Get your ego on your body's sleep-needs side, and make sure you (usually) get enough sleep! If you truly want energy, don't underestimate the supreme importance of sufficient sleep!

Our culture downplays our natural sleep needs. Don't let society mislead you, here. If you want energy and health, don't sleep-deprive yourself day-after-day-after-day!

If you have to take a daily nap (Energy Tool #61) to get your 8 to 9 hours/day of sleep, do it! Or use Soothing, Restful Mantra Meditation (Energy Tool #52); that will help a lot here, too.

Of course, once in a while you might need to shorten your sleep needs a bit, in an emergency. But don't make this a habit, or you'll be losing a lot of energy and even healthiness, with any habitual sleep insufficiency or neglect!

Energy Tool

#80. Smoking: Stop Fast (Or Cut Down)

It's fairly well known these days that smoking cigarettes tends to diminish your health, and your energy too. Yet, cigarettes are very addictive and quite hard to stop!

But, if you really want to stop or cut down smoking (in order to have more energy), I've written another book (available from Lulu.com or Amazon) entitled "Stop Smoking Fast. 15 Methods that Actually Work, Plus 45 Mini-Methods", by Gary Pickler.

Your smoking will definitely be done with, if you read this book. Pick a suitable method to stop, and apply it. Do it, if you truly want to stop or cut down on smoking cigarettes, to then have lots more energy!

Energy Tool

#81. Steam Sweat In Shower

Many people have accumulated numerous toxins in their body, that can be sweated out of their skin, in a hot shower. Once these toxins are removed, you'll eventually have more energy, once you replenish yourself with nutritious foods afterward.

Instructions For A Steam-Sweating Shower:

(1) Cover your head with a towel dipped in cold water, and then squeezed out. It's a sort of "turban" you wear, to protect your brain from the extreme heat.

(2) Take as hot a shower as your skin can possibly stand. As you do this, scrub your skin with a wash rag and a soap that absolutely does not clog your skin's pores! Don't use any soap with deodorant or additives or chemicals, which all clog your skin's pores, which reduces sweating! Recommended is either a natural soap (see Energy Tool #76) or Ivory soap.

(3) Stand in the shower's hot water, after washing off the soap, for about 10 minutes, as you sweat and sweat and sweat! (It's possible for you to be sitting on a small stool here, instead of standing.) Have the hot water run down your back, as you stand or sit.

(4) After 10 minutes, turn the shower's water to cold (or as cold as you can stand it).

(5) Scrub yourself off a second time, with the wash rag and soap, to remove all the oily sweat accumulated on the surface of your skin (that will harden, and feel terrible, if not scrubbed off in this second wash-rag scrubbing).

(6) Step out of your "steam-sweating" shower, dry off, and feel how good your skin feels, and how much better you feel emotionally (from sweating out all those toxins and washing them away).

(7) Drink plenty of water (filtered water is best), and eat some nourishing natural foods to rebuild blood-nutrient levels. (You may feel a little "tipsy" after all the sweating, because the sweating may have reduced the nutrients along with the toxins.)

(8) Don't drive your car for a while, until you feel completely stabilized and back to normal again.

Note. Do not do this steam-sweating shower if you have a weak heart! High water-temperatures in a shower, with a long session of sweating, can overly strain a weak heart.

Energy Tool

#82. Stretch And Shake

One of the best ways to have more energy (and feel much better too) is to stretch and shake. Now, there are plenty of "advanced stretching" books about this on the internet, and plenty of courses to take also, but this simple "intermediate" method works well for me, and just might work for you too:

Instructions:

(1) Bend each of your 10 fingers backward (as it hurts a bit from the stretching) back about 4" or maybe more, or until you feel the amount of pain indicates you could almost be starting to damage your finger. In other words, stretch each finger back to its "healthy limit" of stretching, without any threat of damage. Experiment with this, "staying on the safe side", with this "backward stretching" of your 10 fingers.

(2) Repeat this bending-backward-stretching with your wrists, elbows, and shoulder joints (safely). Then do this with your toes, ankles, knees, and hip joints (safely). With shoulder joints and hip joints, I slowly twirl them around in a circle, first clockwise, then counterclockwise.

(3) Standing, move your head around in a circle (safely) to gently stretch your neck. Then, let your body "twist, circle, and stretch", kind of spontaneously and randomly (safely). You can either dance around a bit, or just stand there, as you stretch your body like this (safely).

(4) Now, still standing, shake back and forth (gently, if you need to) each part of your body. Shake each arm. Then shake each leg (as your weight is on the other leg). Safely, grab hold of something for balance here, if necessary. Then, with slightly bent knees, sort of vibrate and "shake around" your whole body (including your head, a little, too).

Doesn't all this feel great?

Afterward, do your muscles now all feel a bit more relaxed, from all this stretching and shaking? Good!

Usually, I need to repeat this entire sequence about 5 times, until I'm feeling utter and complete relaxation (and increased energy) in my body, from this stretching and shaking. (Total time for all this is only about 10 or 15 minutes.)

Try it!

P.S. Whenever my body feels an extreme need for stretching, I find that, instead, I am very dehydrated, and I need to drink lots and lots of water! After abundant water, I no longer feel the need for stretching (see Energy Tool #96).

Energy Tool

#83. Strongest Muscles Press Method

There is a system called "Bodynamics", invented by Peter Bernhardt in Oakland and Berkeley, California, around 1980. For a literature list, see

- https://www.bodynamic.com/blog/scientific-validation-of-the-bodynamic-system/

The essence of this system is that all the muscles in your entire body's Muscular System can be organized into seven groups as:

- (Category 1) Very Strong
- (Category 2) Strong
- (Category 3) Above Average in Strength
- (Category 4) Average Strength
- (Category 5) Below Average in Strength
- (Category 6) Weak
- (Category 7) Very Weak

Bodynamics was intended to go beyond Wilhelm Reich's system of healing so-called muscular armoring, in order to even more effectively heal any chronic tension in the muscles.

However, this author has found by experience that when massaging and pressing Category 1 – Very Strong muscles, then great energy and willpower is produced.

This author's strongest muscles turned out to be the arm's biceps, along with the trapezius muscles (they're along the top of the shoulders, from the neck to the shoulder blades, and are used to shrug the shoulders). Whenever a noxious chore arose, this author would vigorously massage both biceps and both trapezius muscles. The resultant energy and great strength of will that resulted would be used to plunge into the odious chore and "do it anyway".

A shortcut to finding your strongest muscles can be massaging the muscles you've made strongest in sports or weight-lifting, and seeing how it makes you feel when these (or any other) muscles are massaged!

I sometimes also press the pectorals (chest muscles) or front deltoids (upper shoulder muscles) for great bursts of energy and willpower.

So, this is how it could work: whenever low energy strikes, quickly massage or press your strongest muscles, to energize yourself. Have this strategy all worked out in advance, so that when low energy strikes, you can quickly deflect it!

Energy Tool

#84. Sugar: Stop (Or Cut Down)

Most people find they get quite a bit more energy when they cut way down on sugar.

Many, many books have been written about why sugar is bad for your health, etc. But it's very hard to stop, because sugar is practically an addiction!

However, these two books will genuinely help you to stop. First is Dufty's very entertaining book "Sugar Blues", which helps you to totally understand why sugar is a harmful drug that must be stopped! Second is my brief 36-page book "Stop Sugar Craving Fast", by Gary Pickler, that gives a quick and easy way to effortlessly end all sugar craving (fast).

With much less sugar intake, your energy should noticeably increase, especially when combined with a better, more nutritious diet!

Energy Tool

#85. Sunshine And Sun-Bathing

It's very well known about the benefits of being in sunshine (without overdoing it and getting sunburn). Sunlight uplifts you emotionally, and makes you feel much more enthusiastic and energized (than on a cloudy or rainy day).

Take full advantage of the healthy energy of sunlight. Perhaps the right amount of sunbathing every day is 20 minutes facing the sun (with eyes closed, of course, or even wearing dark glasses). And then another 20 minutes facing away from the sun, so that sunlight will hit the entire back of you (when perhaps wearing a swimsuit).

Sunbathing for only 20 minutes (front), then 20 minutes (back) shouldn't require any suntan lotion, but if you think you really might need the lotion, put it on (obviously).

Try to regularly energize yourself with sunshine, in moderation and balance, whenever you can. You'll be glad you did!

Energy Tool

#86. Superfoods

There exist today several superfoods, plus vitamin and mineral supplements, which supply you with enormous amounts of nutritional energy!

Every day, I take the following supplements:

(1) Raw Meal Protein Powder (5 heaping teaspoons),

(2) Sunwarrior Protein Powder (2 heaping teaspoons),

(3) Sunwarrior Super Greens (1 level teaspoon),

(4) Blue-green algae/spirulina/chlorella mix (1 level teaspoon),

(5) Reishi Mushroom ("Gano Ultra" label on bottle, 4 powder capsules),

(6) Cordyceps Mushroom (4 powder capsules),

(7) Vitamin A (25,000 IU),

(8) Vitamin B Complex (all eleven B vitamins must be in it, 1 capsule),

(9) Vitamin C (500 mg buffered with magnesium, 1 capsule),

(10) Vitamin E (400 IU, 1 capsule),

(11) Vitamins K and K-2,

(12) Multi Minerals (3 tablets, call 1-866-293-3367 to order).

All these superfoods and supplements can be found on the internet and ordered.

I know this is quite a bit of supplements, but it makes me feel (physically and emotionally) absolutely great! I also eat a nutritious, balanced diet, of mostly natural and organically grown foods, bought at a nearby health food store.

People of low energy often have very poor nutrition. When nutrition is greatly improved, often energy increases.

I greatly encourage anyone without enough energy to try a balanced, nutritional diet at some health food store in their vicinity, and to start taking all (or most) of the supplements that I've listed above.

Then, you'll feel nutritionally super!

Energy Tool

#87. T'ai Chi, Spontaneously

In the far distant Chinese past, perhaps seven thousand years ago, it was Chinese intuitives, mystics, artists, and inventors who originally created what today is called T'ai Chi Ch'uan. It is also said that movements of animals were incorporated into the movements. Thus, when you learn T'ai Chi Ch'uan today, you're supposed to rigorously and painstakingly "copycat" what the original intuitive people put together.

But, think about this! Why do we need to mindlessly (like an automaton) follow blindly what some 7,000-year-old Chinese men invented? Why can't we also creatively invent a sequence of spontaneous movements that works for us? They did! Why can't we also do the same, along with a much smaller amount of imitating, from watching present-day T'ai Chi DVDs?

I've experimented (abundantly) with doing my own (totally-spontaneous) version of T'ai Chi, and it works incredibly well, in relaxing me and putting my mind at peace. I invite you to do the same!

See what this means! You don't have to laboriously take a lengthy T'ai Chi class, or pay (usually) high fees. If you're quite intuitive, just spontaneously allow your body to do those "slow flowing movements" that produce the calmness, relaxation, and serenity that your soul seeks. And, if you're only "semi-intuitive", then put on a T'ai Chi DVD, but only approximately follow along with the movements according to your tastes and desires! You'll still feel quite energized afterward, from these "slow flowing movements" that calm your spirit, relax your body, and soothe your soul.

Try it! After all, it's far better to enjoyably do your own version of T'ai Chi, than none at all, due to its extreme difficulty and expense!

Energy Tool

#88. T'ai Chi Chih

There is a much simplified version of T'ai Chi Ch'uan called T'ai Chi Chih. Justin F. Stone, the originator of this system, wrote a book "T'ai Chi Chih". It has 1 pose and 19 simple-to-do movements, and their energetic, relaxing, and calming benefits.

You can either get this book on the internet, or find DVDs available on T'ai Chi Chih.

Try these simple movements. They really energize, relax, and calm you significantly!

For more information, see

*   https://justinstonetcc.com/

P.S. It's also possible to first do some T'ai Chi Chih, then follow up with some "T'ai Chi, Spontaneously" (Energy Tool #87).

Energy Tool

#89. Talk To Body Parts And Ask What's Wrong

There is a book available on the internet entitled "Conversations With The Body", by Robyn Welch. This book tells her story of how she became a "medical intuitive", by developing her ability to "psychically talk" with the body parts of sick people to ask, "What's wrong?"

In her book, Welch guides you to develop your own ability to "talk" to your own body parts, in order to most effectively heal them! Welch says that all body parts can be conversed with, once you learn how (with practice). Also, this communication with your body parts will make them feel more befriended and appreciated, so that these body parts will work harder for you! Thus, you'll have more energy from this.

By no longer neglecting and ignoring your body parts, this communication with them will facilitate healing of these body parts, which will result in much more energy in your entire body, eventually.

Get Welch's book, read it, then try all this. It works!

Energy Tool

#90. Tongue Touches Roof Of Mouth Technique

In Mantak Chia's book "Awaken Healing Energy Through The Tao", he explains a very energizing technique that he calls "circulating energy in the completed microcosmic orbit".

The (6,000 years old) Chinese Medicine System describes 14 "meridians" of circulating chi-energy in the human body. Two of these very-energizing meridians are called the "Governor Meridian/ Energy Stream", and the "Conception Meridian/Energy Stream". (Diagrams of these two powerful meridians can be viewed on the internet.) The Governor Meridian begins at the base of the trunk, or perineum (halfway between the genitals and the anus). It flows into the tailbone, up the entire spine (back of the body), through the brain, over the top of the head, and then back down to end at the roof of the mouth. The Conception Meridian (or "Functional" Meridian) also begins at the perineum, but flows upward along the front of the body, past the digestive organs, heart, and throat, to end at the bottom of the mouth.

When your tongue reaches up to touch the roof of your mouth, it connects these two powerful meridians. Your tongue thus acts as a "switch", completing this powerful energizing circuit (called the completed microcosmic orbit)!

Your tongue, when connecting this bodily energy circuit, allows powerful energy to flow in a circle, up the spine, over and around your head, and then back down the front of your body. It becomes an energy loop! Vital energy then circulates past your major organs to give all your cells plenty of chi-energy to function energetically at their very best!

Relaxing bodily tension helps greatly, too, when using your tongue as a "switch" to circulate energy with these two powerful meridians (since bodily tension tends to block and inhibit meridian-flowing energy).

The Governor Meridian is mostly Yang energy, while the Conception Meridian is mostly Yin energy. By connecting them with your "tongue switch", you not only energize your body, but you tend to "Yin-Yang" balance yourself, too!

All this is fully explained in much more detail in Mantak Chia's book "Awaken Healing Energy Through The Tao", starting with pages 1 to 8, and then throughout the rest of the book. In fact, the front cover has a diagram that illustrates this whole process (that you can view on your cell-phone or computer by searching on Amazon for this book)!

Anyway, try it! While sitting, relax your entire body as much as possible, while touching your tongue to the roof of your mouth. Visualize and feel meridian energy come up your spine, go around your head, come down to your mouth, through your tongue, then down along the front of your body to where it started. Doesn't it make you feel calm, centered, grounded in your body, and more energized and balanced, too? This technique greatly helps to connect your mind with your body, to allow you to "feel one, and at peace". It even seems (amazingly!) to connect the two hemispheres of your brain more, I've discovered.

Consider buying Mantak Chia's book, and learning all this thoroughly, if you're drawn to this "two-meridians-connecting-through-the-tongue-switch" way of meditating into a "peace-feeling energized oneness".

Pressing Lips Tightly Together Technique

My father (a military officer) had enormous energy and willpower to work at his tough job and to be constantly fixing everything around the house. I noticed he was often pressing his lips very tightly together, which would have the effect of connecting the two meridians through his compressed lips, and would also tend to jam the top and bottom of his mouth together with the tongue (a bit) squashed between them (connecting the two meridians). It seems he (unknowingly) found a way to powerfully connect the two meridians, through his compressed lips and clamped-shut mouth! When I've tried this, it does seem to give me a burst of "super willpower", but with "fed-up anger" mixed in there, too! Experiment with this technique, if you're curious. It's also possible to shove the tongue forward against your front teeth (upper and lower front teeth), while tightly closing your mouth (but without too much lip pressing). Then, the front of your tongue connects the top and bottom of your mouth, and thus connects the two meridians in this way.

Try playing around with all this, and finding your own unique way of powerfully connecting the two meridians, using the most effective positionings of your tongue, lips, mouth, and possibly even sucked-in cheeks, too!

Energy Tool

#91. Tree Hugging

Trees are full of energy, and you actually do get energy from them when you hug them! I realize that our society teaches you to be skeptical about this, and says that "tree huggers" are "flaky hippies", etc. But still, tree hugging actually does give you more energy, and the only way to find this out is to keep an open mind and try it! Also, you know that if it doesn't work for you (personally, as an individual) you can just curse, kick the tree, and stomp angrily away. Right? (Just kidding.)

To start, experimentally pick a tree that's

(1) big,

(2) healthy looking, and

(3) isolated and away from people,

so that you won't be embarrassed if some stranger comes across you "weirdly" hugging the tree. Incidentally, if that ever happens, then immediately stop hugging the tree, smile, and say to the stranger: "Ha, ha. I read in some book about 'tree hugging', and I thought I'd give it a try. Ha, ha!" The stranger will probably just politely smile back at you, and continue walking past (if you're not dressed like a hippie, in which case you could get beaten up as a suspected communist—just kidding again). Then, when they're out of sight, resume hugging your tree experimentally.

Tips on this:

(1) Don't hug small trees because they have little or no energy to give you.

(2) Don't hug unhealthy-looking trees, or you'll receive sickly or unhealthy energy from them! (I've had this happen. It sucks.)

(3) Before hugging a tree, closely inspect it for ants, ticks, or other bugs.

(4) Lastly, don't get freaked out if, somehow, it seems that the tree starts communicating with you intuitively in some way! This has happened to me, and I still don't know if the "message" was really from the tree, or from my own unconscious mind, just pretending it was coming from the tree. Anyway, just write down the "message" afterward, and decide yourself as to its source (or whether to pay attention to it or not). Who knows? The tree (or your unconscious mind) may have something important for you to listen to!

For what it's worth, one big, powerful tree "seemed" to ask me to tell humanity that

(1) trees are just as highly evolved (in Higher Consciousness) in the plant kingdom, as humans are in the animal kingdom. Thus, trees (especially big ones) should be much more respected, and shouldn't be looked upon as just something to be sawed down, to be turned into lumber to build houses with, etc.

Also, I was told that

(2) trees all over our planet are in telepathic communication with each other. Okay! Here, in writing these words, I've honored that tree's request, if the request really was from the tree and not from my own unconscious mind!

Anyway, try it! Experimentally hug a big, healthy-looking, bug-free tree for at least 10 minutes and experience any results you get. Very likely, it won't be the last tree you ever hug!

P.S. You won't turn into any kind of "flaky hippie" (or commie) by doing this. Instead, you'll be a courageous experimenter who has the guts to try new, innovative things!

Energy Tool

#92. Tryptophan-Rich Foods Eating

(or Tryptophan caps, or 5-HTP)

Tryptophan is an amino acid that tends to make you feel high, lifting you out of any depression. Certain foods are tryptophan-rich, and serve to abundantly supply you with this mood-lifting and energizing tryptophan. High dietary tryptophan gives significantly less depression and irritability, and decreased anxiety.

Category-1 tryptophan-rich foods "A" (612-900 mg per 6 oz serving): tuna (canned, but the ocean is incredibly polluted, including with radiation, so I wouldn't advise eating tuna more than once a week), pumpkin seeds, squash, pumpkin pie, milk, yogurt, kefir, ice cream, cottage cheese, beef, pork chops, turkey.

Category-2 tryptophan-rich foods "B" (416-592 mg per 6 oz serving): tofu (firm), salmon, cheddar cheese, cheese (in general), chicken, fish (in general), duck, cashews, pistachio nuts, soybeans (boiled), soy milk.

Category-3 tryptophan-rich foods "C" (200-390 mg per 6 oz serving): nuts, almonds, walnuts, peanuts, seeds, Swiss cheese, eggs, white beans (large), red kidney beans.

Category-4 tryptophan-rich foods "D" (110-185 mg per cup or 6 oz serving): pinto beans, black beans, lentils, oats, bread (whole wheat), chocolate.

Category-5 tryptophan-rich foods "E" (17-41 mg per 6 oz serving): zucchini, sweet potatoes, bananas, yams, spinach, lettuce.

Category-6 tryptophan-rich foods "F" (very little): honey, sugar, rice, potatoes, corn.

Experiment with eating these foods ("A's" and "B's" have by far the most tryptophan) to find out which ones make you feel good and energized most, with their richness in tryptophan!

Health food stores have a supplement called 5-HTP (5-hydroxytryptophan). This 5-HTP undergoes a transformation (in your body) to become tryptophan (supplying you with it).

Before the 1970s, it used to be possible to buy capsules of tryptophan at health food stores. This probably is still possible at some places, or over the internet. Check on it.

You might need to include (a bit) of the rest of the 22 amino acids, with the (larger) amount of tryptophan you take, since there's some evidence that all the 22 amino acids tend to work together.

Anyway, the improved mood that you get from tryptophan will result in greater energy!

Energy Tool

#93. Troubles Spill To Pet, Stuffed Animal, Or Photo Of Past Friend

We all have a lot of gripes, complaints, troubles, shop talk, gossip, reasonings-out, and just plain talk, on and on, that fervently wants to spill out of our mouth! Yes, we all need someone to talk to, about all our "stuff". Right? But we've probably already poured out most of this talk onto all our friends, spouse, children, or relatives. In fact, it's already been so much that they don't really want to hear any more of it! And yet, we still have a big back load that hasn't all quite been said!

Of course, we can spill out all our troubles on Facebook or various internet sites, but this just isn't as rewarding as a face-to-face talk-out. Right?

Firstly, we don't actually require another human being to satisfy our face-to-face talk-out needs! We can talk-it-all-out with our dog or cat, as we pet them. (And it's so wonderful that they don't talk back.) Secondly, we can talk (as long as we want) to a teddy bear, other stuffed animal, or doll (etc.). Thirdly, we can color-xerox-enlarge a photo of a past friend (or even a current friend), paste the xerox to cardboard, and cut it out, so that it's as big as, and closely resembles the friend's face. Then we can talk openly to this "friendly face" that we've created here. (Try it—this really works!) You can even talk to trees, your car, or even to your computer or TV set!

Anyway, by verbally releasing all our troubles in these ways, we'll more thoroughly "talk-it-out", be much more relaxed and happy, and thus have more energy!

P.S. Think also of how much money we'll save, by not paying some counselor or shrink, to "listen to it all!" Instead, we can put all these hundreds of dollars in the bank, to pay for our next super-adventurous travel excursion!

Energy Tool

#94. Turmeric Force

This supplement, Turmeric Force, put out by New Chapter (on the internet) gives you a daily megadose of turmeric, which gives you more energy due to turmeric being a strong and effective anti-oxidant. Also, turmeric has lots of silica, a very needed trace mineral (that most people are quite deficient in). Take 1 capsule daily, with a meal. It's quite effective in energizing you!

Gary Pickler

Energy Tool

#95. Vitamin C Intravenous Injections (For COVID-19 Help, Possible Cure)

I first read about intravenous injections of vitamin C (that kill viruses in the bloodstream) in a book "Let's Eat Right To Keep Fit" by Adelle Davis[1]. On page 136, line 17, it's said that a doctor injected 50 to 100 grams of vitamin C (50,000 to 100,000 milligrams) in a 5-percent dextrose solution, accompanied by administering lots of vitamin C by mouth, too. Patients hopelessly ill with virus pneumonia often recovered after a single injection of vitamin C, it's stated here.

In this same book, on page 131, lines 30-31, administering vitamin C by injection is mentioned too, to successfully treat meningitis, encephalitis, virus pneumonia, and scarlet fever, even in patients who had not been expected to live! Also on page 132, line 1, line 9, line 20, line 24, and line 34, vitamin C injection is mentioned as being practically a "miracle drug", in quickly reducing fever and successfully healing many virus-caused diseases! Get this book and read about all this, to confirm all this, if you want to!

A friend from Toronto, Canada said that he knew of a pharmacy there that sold legal, over-the-counter vitamin C injecting equipment, with instructions. Perhaps all this can be ordered over the internet, along with trustworthy instructions?

I absolutely do not understand why doctors in hospitals are so ignorant of the enormous disease-fighting powers of vitamin C injections, when Adelle Davis's book came out in 1954 (68 years ago!) Are doctors not told about vitamin C injections in medical school, and are thus ignorant? Especially, when they attribute the cause of so many diseases to viruses (little affected by antibiotics) killing so many people? Ask yourself what kind of doctor-craziness and hospital-craziness is going on, here.

I sincerely hope people will quickly and seriously look into this vitamin C injection cure, and obtain a doctor who is willing to do it for you, if COVID-19 or any other viral disease is caught! Obviously, preparations to do this vitamin C injection cure must be set up now, as a standby treatment plan, that can be immediately launched whenever COVID-19, or any other viral disease, is caught. Right?

Also, how safe is it, to actually inject vitamin C into yourself? Is a doctor needed for this, or not? Research this, and plan ahead, because it seems that most hospitals and doctors in 2022 are totally ignorant of

1   The book can be borrowed online, here:
*   https://archive.org/details/letseatrighttoke0000davi

this "miracle cure" of vitamin C injection!

Incidentally, it's possible to combine vitamin C intravenous injections with colloidal silver (which also very effectively kills viruses). See Energy Tool #24.

Besides injecting vitamin C, it's also possible to take (by mouth) "Ester C". "Ester C" is massive amounts of vitamin C taken by mouth, but combined with either magnesium or calcium, so that these large amounts of vitamin C (taken orally) won't upset the stomach or intestines. Lots of "Ester C" taken orally also is very effective in killing off viral infections. Research and read up on all this! (Be sure to be near a bathroom when taking lots of "Ester C", because it can often be an extremely powerful laxative that will have you running to the toilet.)

Additionally, there are many other antiviral herbs, substances, and drugs, too. Some of these herbs are available from Chinese Medicine practitioners and acupuncturists. Search the internet for the rest. You'll be glad that you did!

Energy Tool

#96. Water Stops Energy Loss Resulting From Dehydration

In our rat-race, ultra-citified environment, we're often dehydrated, without even knowing it! Insufficient water can often cause stress and bodily fatigue.

So, keep up your fluid intake, daily, to avoid this possible dehydration. Drinking six tall glasses of water every day should be enough. Water helps to lubricate and detox all the organs of your body.

Drinking filtered water seems best, in order to filter out any "unhealthy stuff", in the water.

It might be a bit of a strain at first, drinking so much water (six tall glasses) every day. If you're not used to so much water, then gradually work up to six tall glasses per day.

Eventually, you should notice your daily energy increasing, from drinking sufficient water each day.

Highly recommended here, is the excellent book "Your Body's Many Cries For Water", by F. Batmanghelidj, M.D.

Energy Tool

#97. Whistle Or Sing Your Most Energizing Song Or Tune

We've all been inspired and energized by music! And, most of us have our very favorite tunes. Well, it doesn't really matter how skillfully you can sing, hum, or whistle (you'll get better with practice anyway). The point here is to start whistling or singing your favorite songs or tunes to psychologically and emotionally energize yourself!

It works! You know it does by how you feel when your favorite tunes are heard on the radio, TV, computer, or while watching a movie (etc.). So, start this energizing process by whistling or singing yourself (instead of relying so much on "outside sources"). Or, perhaps your intuition can just "pop" the right tune into your head, that most outstandingly facilitates every life situation you're in? Try it!

A more advanced level of this is to have a collection of tunes to sing, to stimulate yourself for specific activities. You can have tunes for working (in general), tunes for specific jobs to do, tunes to facilitate socializing with your friends, tunes to meditate by, tunes for travelling, and tunes for easing depression, anger, anxiety, stress, or fatigue!

Start using your favorite music today, for energy and lots more. Since it's so easy to just start listening to your favorite tunes (even in your car), this is such a convenient energy tool to always have right on hand!

Energy Tool

#98. Wrist Tendons Stroke-Massage

The fingers don't really stop at your knuckles! If you look at an anatomy chart, the tendons of these fingers go through the hands to the wrists, then from there down the forearm's topside, to the elbow. So, in a way, our "fingers" are really about 1 1/2 feet long!

Our fingers are used so extensively in the modern world, that the tendons attached to them often become quite stressed and even painful. These upper-forearm tendons, so over-used on computer keyboards, etc., often become quite afflicted, even to the point of "carpal-tunnel" problems.

The solution is to regularly stroke and massage these topside forearm tendons, in the most effective way. This energy tool will show you how:

Directions:

(1) Put a little coconut oil on the topside of your left forearm (this is optional; you can still do all this without oil.)

(2) Now, massage along the forearm's topside, from your wrist to your elbow.

(3) Try using your knuckles (the big ones that join your fingers to your hands). Or, try doing it with the heel of your right hand. Or, even, with the side of your right hand. It's best not to use the right hand's fingers at all, or you'll be straining your fingers again (which is exactly what you're trying to heal!) Experimentally, find which part of your right hand makes your left (topside) forearm feel the best, in your massage strokes.

(4) Try massaging up the forearm in slightly sideways (45-degree-angle) strokes. With this, you're sort of massaging diagonally across all the finger tendons. Doesn't this 45-degree-angle massage feel even better?

(5) Now switch hands and forearms, so that your left hand is massaging the topside of the right forearm, in the same way.

Don't your forearm tendons feel just super after all this? Begin to do this regularly, so that your forearms can feel these pleasurable sensations on a regular basis.

Try it!

P.S. You can also do this while sitting in a hot bathtub, using soap on your forearm's topsides, instead of coconut oil!

P.P.S. Using the Roller Massager (Energy Tool #74) to roll along (and massage) your forearm tendons, is pure ecstasy. Put the *heel* of your other hand (not the fingers) on top of the Roller Massager's two balls, to press it down onto the tendons, as you roll it up and down your arm. You'll feel "forearm heaven"!

Energy Tool

#99. Yawning For Energy

Yawning pumps energy into you whenever you're tired! Many people have found themselves yawning automatically when they start becoming sleepy or tired. Afterward, they may even feel slightly more energetic, after the yawn. But usually people regard yawning as an automatic reaction, which "happens" to them (instead of their choosing it). Well, it doesn't always have to be this way!

You can begin to deliberately yawn, when you need more energy! Just open your mouth wide, perhaps tilt your head back a bit, and attempt a deliberate yawn. (Just let your body do it, after you deliberately "jump-start" it.) You'll find that the extra air you breathe in, deeply, helps give you significantly more energy. In fact, the "act of yawning" actually is a pumping into yourself of more energy, which the very wise teacher Gurdjieff explains (in great detail) on page 235 of Ouspensky's book "In Search of the Miraculous".

Yes! From now on, whenever you want some instant, quick, physical (and mental) energy, try deliberate yawning, and even try breathing in and out deeply, several times, with your wide-open yawning mouth! It's very refreshing. Also, you feel so much better, after the yawn!

However, since this extra energy comes from your "energy reserves" (as Gurdjieff explains) it's probably a good idea to limit yourself to perhaps twenty yawns a day (about once every hour?) so as not to drain too much these deeper energy reserves that your yawning is tapping.

(Don't over-do it, with "too much of a good thing", here.) Doesn't this make sense? Be careful with this "free energy" tool!

Anyway, enjoy this tool of yawning for energy, throughout your day, whenever needed, up to (perhaps) twenty yawns a day.

P.S. Some people, when they start yawning in the evening, just overwhelmingly want to go to bed, quickly. If this is your pattern, you can still try "yawning for more energy" in the morning or early afternoon, only. Experiment with this! Perhaps you can only be an "early bird yawner-for-more-energy"!

Energy Tool

#100. Yogis, Gurus, And Psychic Healers Contacting

A good, trusted friend of mine (named David) told me of how, after crashing badly in a motorcycle accident, many of his bones were all disconnected and in very bad shape. The doctors were all shaking their heads and telling him that he'd never walk again, etc. But he prayed fervently and frequently to the first guru of Yogananda in his book, "Autobiography of a Yogi". (A picture of his first guru is in this book.) Miraculously, his bones slowly began to knit together again, until eventually he was completely healed. As usual, in these kinds of cases, the doctors were "utterly amazed".

I had another friend named Cathy, who recently had a bad ear infection. She went to a Christian Science Healing Practitioner. It worked, her ear healed, and she has never had any trouble with that ear again.

I, myself, was once in a state of extremely low physical energy (40 years ago, before knowing any of these Energy Tools). Hearing of a healing group (at a distance), I contacted them, and asked for healing energy. I received it, and my health and energy level significantly improved. It really worked! I insisted on sending them $50, even though they usually worked for free.

The point here is that psychic healing (by practitioners) can actually work! "Resurrection" with Ellen Burstyn, is a movie about this topic, available on DVD and BluRay.

If you need energy, or have something that needs healing, it really might be worth your while to seek out some psychic healing practitioner and give them a try (as long as they're not the type charging a lot of money, to possibly scam you). Be open-minded about this, and investigate it! Perhaps even try praying fervently to the same guru that I mentioned in the first paragraph, above!

Energy Tool

#101. Way Of Random Choice

This is for those who can't make up their mind of which of the 100 Energy Tools to try first!

Perhaps all these Energizing Methods are just too overwhelming for some people. Well, instead of just throwing your arms in the air, in confusion and indecision, maybe you could let a "playing card and coin combo" decide which of the 100 Energy Tools to try first!

Instructions:

(1) From an ordinary deck of 52 playing cards, take out any jokers, and also remove the 2 of clubs and the three of clubs, so that there are now just 50 cards left.

(2) Get any regular coin that has a clear "head" on one side, and a "tail" on the other side.

(3) Shuffle the deck of cards, draw out a random card, and flip the coin. Then, match up your drawn card and the heads-or-tails result (of the coin) to the list below. You now have your first random choice of an Energy Tool!

(4) If you like this random choice of an Energy Tool, then go ahead and (experimentally) start using it, to energize yourself!

(5) But if you don't really like what has randomly come up, then go back to step (3) and try it all over again, with another drawn card and coin flip.

(6) Keep drawing a random card and flipping the coin until you get an Energy Tool that you like enough to actually begin doing, starting today!

Randomly drawn playing card (and coin flip) matched up with the 100 Energy Tools:

SPADE

Spade Ace, Heads → 1. Acupressure Points of Power

Spade Ace, Tails → 2. Aerobic Shape

Spade King, Heads → 3. Air Filter In Home

Spade King, Tails → 4. Alcohol Minimize Or Stop

Spade Queen, Heads → 5. Ally Sub-Self Method

Spade Queen, Tails → 6. Aromatherapy: Pine, Basil, or Patchouli

Spade Jack, Heads → 7. Art Project Initiate

Spade Jack, Tails → 8. B-Vitamin Energy

Spade 10, Heads → 9. Back Roller Massager (or Theracane)

Spade 10. Tails → 10. Bad-Back Exercises

Spade 9, Heads → 11. Biorhythms

Spade 9. Tails → 12. Book Of Internal Exercises

Spade 8, Heads → 13. Brain Gym Exercises

Spade 8. Tails → 14. Brain Relax

Spade 7, Heads → 15. Canine Yoga

Spade 7. Tails → 16. Chi From Hands Into Food

Spade 6, Heads → 17. Chi From Hands Into Organs

Spade 6. Tails → 18. Chi Gong (Chinese Yoga)

Spade 5, Heads → 19. Chi-Nei-Tsang

Spade 5. Tails → 20. Chinese Dietary Therapy

Spade 4, Heads → 21. Chinese Tonic Pills

Spade 4.Tails → 22. Chiropractic-Towel-Under-Spine Technique

Spade 3, Heads → 23. Circadian Rhythms

Spade 3. Tails → 24. Colloidal Silver (For COVID-19 Help)

Spade 2, Heads → 25. Color Therapy Glasses (Green)

Spade 2. Tails → 26. Color: Wear Your Favorite Color

HEART

Heart Ace Heads → 27. Crying Out Woes To Re-Energize

Heart Ace Tails → 28. Dance Out Stressful Emotions

Heart King Heads → 29. Deep Breathing For More Oxygen

Heart King Tails → 30. Diet (Healthiest)

Heart Queen Heads → 31. Dual Brain Psychology

Heart Queen Tails → 32. $E = M{\cdot}c$, not $E = M{\cdot}J^2$

Heart Jack Heads → 33. Ear Acupressure Point Massage

Heart Jack Tails → 34. Earth Power Spots

Heart 10 Heads → 35. Enema Hose In Shower

Heart 10 Tails → 36. Ester C (For COVID-19 Help)

Heart 9 Heads → 37. Favorite Healing Meal To Fix

Heart 9 Tails → 38. Five-Minute Massage Of 30 Muscles

Heart 8 Heads → 39. Foods (Very Nutritious To Eat)

Heart 8 Tails → 40. Ginseng

Heart 7 Heads → 41. Hands Clasp

Heart 7 Tails → 42. Hatha Yoga

Heart 6 Heads → 43. Hot Bath (Invigorating)

Heart 6 Tails → 44. HSO Probiotics

Heart 5 Heads → 45. Indian Head Massage (Of Scalp)

Heart 5 Tails → 46. Isometrics

Heart 4 Heads → 47. Jin Shin Do Acupressure Point Massage

Heart 4 Tails → 48. Laughing For Energy

Heart 3 Heads → 49. Longan Fruit Heart Tonic

Heart 3 Tails → 50. Lymph Massage

Heart 2 Heads → 51. Massage Of Joints

Heart 2 Tails → 52. Meditation (Soothing, Restful, With Mantra)

DIAMOND

Diamond Ace Heads → 53. Mega-Mag Supplement

Diamond Ace Tails → 54. Meridian Stroking For Energy

Diamond King Heads → 55. Mini-Rebounder

Diamond King Tails → 56. Minimize (Or Stop) Caffeine

Diamond Queen Heads → 57. Minimize (Or Stop) Drugs

Diamond Queen Tails → 58. Moonlight (Reversed With Mirror) Soul Healing

Diamond Jack Heads → 59. Mushrooms Of Power

Diamond Jack Tails → 60. Nam Myoho Renge Kyo

Diamond 10 Heads → 61. Naps

Diamond 10 Tails → 62. Nature Walk

Diamond 9 Heads → 63. Ocean Healing (Water Therapy)

Diamond 9 Tails → 64. Ocean Surf Walk And Negative Ion Theorapy

Diamond 8 Heads → 65. Palming Eyes With Hands

Diamond 8 Tails → 66. Peripheral Vision

Diamond 7 Heads → 67. Pow Wow Step

Diamond 7 Tails → 68. Power Crystal Hold

Diamond 6 Heads → 69. Probiotics and Prebiotics

Diamond 6 Tails → 70. Pulling and Swishing Fluid In Your Mouth

Diamond 5 Heads → 71. Reflexology (Feet)

Diamond 5 Tails → 72. Reflexology (Hands)

Diamond 4 Heads → 73. Rocking Chair Power

Diamond 4 Tails → 74. Roller Massager Power

Diamond 3 Heads → 75. Sex

Diamond 3 Tails → 76. Shower With Non-Pore-Clogging Soap

Diamond 2 Heads → 77. Shungite To Stop 5G EMF

Diamond 2 Tails → 78. Slap Lightly Body All Over

CLUB

Club Ace Heads → 79. Sleep Sufficiently

Club Ace Tails → 80. Smoking: Stop Fast (Or Cut Down)

Club King Heads → 81. Steam Sweat In Shower

Club King Tails → 82. Stretch and Shake

Club Queen Heads → 83. Strongest Muscles Press (For More Energy and Willpower)

Club Queen Tails → 84. Sugar: Stop (Or Cut Down)

Club Jack Heads → 85. Sunshine and Sunbathing

Club Jack Tails → 86. Superfoods and Vitamins

Club 10 Heads → 87. T'ai Chi, Spontaneously

Club 10 Tails → 88. T'ai Chi Chih

Club 9 Heads → 89. Talk To Body Parts and Ask What's Wrong?

Club 9 Tails → 90. Tongue Touches Roof Of Mouth Technique

Club 8 Heads → 91. Tree Hugging For Energy

Club 8 Tails → 92. Tryptophan-Rich Foods Eating

Club 7 Heads → 93. Troubles Spill To Pet, Stuffed Animal, Or Photo Of Past Friend

Club 7 Tails → 94. Turmeric Force

Club 6 Heads → 95. Vitamin C Injections (For COVID-19 Help, Possible Cure)

Club 6 Tails → 96. Water (Stops Energy Loss Resulting From Dehydration)

Club 5 Heads → 97. Whistle Or Sing Your Most Energizing Songs Or Tunes

Club 5 Tails → 98. Wrist Tendons Stroke and Massage

Club 4 Heads → 99. Yawning For Energy

Club 4 Tails → 100. Yogis and Psychic Healers Contacting

Club 3 (remove from the deck, and pick another card)

Club 2 (remove from the deck, and pick another card)

Joker (remove from the deck, and pick another card)

More Energy Tools Needed! Please!

I believe that the best way to help people to energize themselves is to provide them with lots and lots of methods that actually work! Then, people can choose the method that works for them, do this method, and be abundantly energized!

If you know of any other effective method that energizes, please let me know of it! Or, if you tried a combination of methods in this book that worked, then please, share it with me and send an email to my email address: garypickler1@gmail.com (don't forget the "1" after my name). Thank you!

When I receive enough methods from you and others, I will get out a second book, "101 More Energy Tools", and all contributors will get a free copy!

Let's get these energizing tools out into the world as fast as we can, to help all those who are overly fatigued and exhausted. Also, if you liked this book, please give it a 5-star review, to encourage others to get it and let it work for them, too! Thank you, thank you, so much!

Starting An "Energizing Group" In Your Area?

It's possible to start a group in your area (by word of mouth and some ads perhaps), of people who would like to come together regularly to energize, reducing their fatigue and exhaustion. This group could help you to keep doing your favorite Energy Tools, with the support of everyone in your group. People in the group can share, socialize, and teach their favorite energizing techniques, to benefit all the others! Does this sound like it might interest you? Consider trying it, perhaps by first starting with some of your friends!